# Human Genetics

## *An Overview*

# Human Genetics

## *An Overview*

**Alice Marcus**

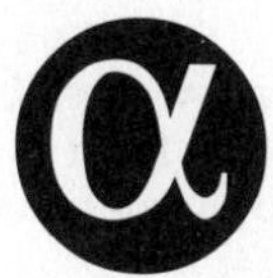

Alpha Science International Ltd.
Oxford, U.K.

**Human Genetics**
An Overview
236 pgs. | 72 figs. | 22 tbls.

**Alice Marcus**
Department of Zoology
Holy Cross College
Trichirappalli



ALPHA SCIENCE INTERNATIONAL LTD.
7200 The Quorum, Oxford Business Park North
Garsington Road, Oxford OX4 2JZ, U.K.

**www.alphasci.com**



ISBN 978-1-84265-574-0

Printed in India

*This book is dedicated to my beloved*

*Marcus*

*Daffy*

*Charles*

# Preface

Human genetics is endlessly fascinating in that genes are the secret of continuity of life. This book is the outcome of experience of more than thirty years of experience in college teaching. I have been planning and doing ground work for a long time to write a book on human genetics including recent developments. The goal in writing this book is to help the reader 'think genetically'.

My intention has been to create a text that would be easy for today's students to learn from a book that focused on concepts rather than mountains of information. A student should learn basic ideas on the subject and the rest comes easy. The fun of learning becomes swamped by a sea of information. To make the concepts more accessible to students, I have trimmed away a lot of details. The internet is blossoming as a teaching resource and no student wants a heavy textbook. Topics have been carefully chosen. It is written in such a way that any reader can get an overall view of human genetics. I believe the treatment of topics is comprehensive and succinct. A good number of examples and figures are included to create interest and to have a better understanding.

At present many Universities and Colleges have introduced Choice Based Credit System (CBCS). Human genetics is included in the list of courses in the curriculum of both Undergraduate and Postgraduate programmes. This book is designed to meet the needs of the shorter, less comprehensive introductory course in human genetics. The brevity of the text more naturally fits the pace of what can be covered in one-semester course. The book has the flexibility to be used in a variety of course formats.

I am deeply indebted to my family members who are God's gift and are a far richer reward than anything in this world. They have become accustomed to the many hours this book draws me away from them. My husband Dr. Marcus Diepen Boominathan, M.Sc., M.Phil., PGDCA., Ph.D, Principal, Bishop Heber College, Trichy, my daughter Miss. Daffodil Marcus, B.Tech., MBA, Project coordinator, Cognizant Foundation, Chennai and my son Dr. Charles Marcus, MBBS, House surgeon, CMC Vellore have provided enormous support without which I could not have completed this task successfully.

My gratitude is due to the publishing team of Narosa publishers, New Delhi.

**Alice Marcus**

# Contents

# List of Tables

# List of Figures

CHAPTER 1

# Introduction to Human Genetics

Genetics is a branch of biology dealing with heredity and variation among related organisms. The word 'genetics' is derived from the Greek word 'genesis' meaning origin. The name **'genetics'** was proposed by Bateson in 1906. Genetics deals with the way the characters are transmitted from one generation to the next. The physical elements, **'genes'** residing in the chromosomes are transmitted from parents to offspring through egg and sperm. Each species has distinguishing features of its own and is maintained generation after generation. Genes respond differently to a wide range of conditions.

The study of transmission of human traits from parent to children is **Human Genetics**. This branch of Genetics deals with the characters that are inherited. These may be physical, mental, normal and abnormal pertaining to an individual or a population. The characters are established and express themselves in an individual during development. A number of factors influence the expression of a trait.

## 1.1 HISTORY OF HUMAN GENETICS

Foundation for the science of Genetics was laid by Gregor Johann Mendel (1866) in nineteenth century. The principles of heredity were derived from his studies on garden pea plant. Prior to Mendel's work some simple pattern of inheritance for common traits like polydactyly and albinism were known.

In 1875 Francis Galton differentiated the effects of environment and heredity. He made quantitative studies and applied mathematical concepts to human heredity.

In 1900 Karl Landsteiner discovered the genetic basis of ABO blood group.

In 1902 Garrod, reported alkaptonuria as an example for Mendelian inheritance.

Sutton and Boveri proposed the chromosome theory of inheritance in 1903.

Bateson named the science of Heredity as 'Genetics' in 1906.

In 1908 Hardy and Weinberg formulated the Hardy Weinberg Law relating gene frequencies and genotype frequencies in randomly mating populations.

In 1908 Nilsson Ehle put forwarded the multiple factor hypothesis.

Garrod developed the concept of 'Inborn errors of metabolism' in 1908.

W. Johansen coined the term 'Gene' in 1909.

In 1940 K.S. Landsteiner and A.S. Wiener discovered Rh factor.

Beadle and Tatum proposed 'one gene – one enzyme hypothesis' in 1941 and elaborated Biochemical Genetics.

Getty Cori and Carl Cori demonstrated the enzyme defect in glycogen storage disease in 1952.

J.D. Watson and F.H.C. Crick proposed the double-helix structure of DNA.

In 1953 Jervis detected the absence of phenylalanine hydroxylase enzyme in PKU.

Allison studied the relationship between malaria and sickle hemoglobin gene in 1954.

Tijo and Leaven in 1956 showed for the first time the diploid number of chromosomes to be 46 in human.

In 1957 Ingram showed the relationship between gene and amino acid sequence. He revealed the difference between normal and sickle hemoglobin in terms of amino acid constitution.

Lejeune and his colleagues identified Downsyndrome then known as Mongoloid idiocy in 1959. They identified the cause to be chromosomal aberration.

In 1959 the role of Y chromosome in determining sex in man was shown by Ford and Jacobs.

In 1961 Jacob and Monad proposed the 'Operon model' for gene regulation.

The Lyon hypothesis was proposed to explain X chromosome inactivation in females by several researchers in 1961.

M.W. Nirenberg and Khorana established the complete genetic code in 1966.

Berg produced the first recombinant DNA in 1972.

In 1976 Y.W. Kan and his co-workers identified polymorphism in beta globin gene to predict sickle cell anemia *in utero*.

Bishop and Varmus demonstrated the protoncogene and oncogene relationship in 1976.

Maxim, Gilbert and Sanger published DNA sequencing techniques in 1977.

Ray White and his colleagues used RFLP as genetic markers to track genetic diseases in 1980.

Lap-Chee mapped cystic fibrosis gene to chromosome 7 in 1983. In the same year the gene for Huntington's disease was located to chromosome 4.

In 1984 Alec Jeffrey developed genetic fingerprinting.

In 1985 Ray and his colleagues identified DMD gene.

Cystic fibrosis gene was cloned in 1989.

Human genome project was launched in 1990.

In 1990 Anderson reported first successful gene therapy in humans.

A rough draft of the human genome map was produced in 1998 showing the locations of more than 30,000 genes.

Human chromosome 22 was the first one to be sequenced in 1999.

Craig Venter and Francis Collins announced first complete draft of the human genome in 2001.

In 2003 Human genome project was successfully completed with 98% of the genome sequenced to 99.99% accuracy.

In 2003 complete sequence of Y chromosome was published.

## 1.2 PROBLEMS IN HUMAN GENETICS STUDY

Most of the information in Genetics is derived from animals and plants. Recently bacteria and viruses have been exploited as genetic tool to study the nature of genetic material and its action in the cell. The basic principles established in the lower group organisms are also applied to human beings. The human is not an ideal creature to genetic study.

Any genetic study should be followed for several generations to determine the transmission of a trait in the members of a family line. The span of human generation is long. So many generations of one family can not be followed in the life time of an investigator. A person can not contribute much to the study of his family, since he may not know the details of his ancestors.

Most of the traits in human do not show clear cut boundaries and are often altered by many factors such as environment, food and behavior (e.g. skin color, height).

Animals and plants can produce large number of offspring in a relatively short period by just a single pair of parents. This is not possible in human.

Any study must involve large sample otherwise sampling error will occur. To minimize the role of chance factors any study must be carried out with large numbers.

An advantage with animal system is that mating or cross may be manipulated. Any kind of cross like between sibs and parents are possible with fruit flies and mice in order to observe how a trait is transmitted. Such manipulations help in determining the purity of a trait.

Since there are so many drawbacks in the use of human in genetic studies, other simpler organisms are used to establish most of the genetic principles. The human has nevertheless been the source of information in establishing the relationship between genes and certain biochemical pathways. The technology explosion enables the utilization of human as a tool in molecular level.

## 1.3 GENETIC DISORDERS AND HEALTH CARE

Genetic studies pertaining to human population inhabiting widely varying ecological conditions provide vital information on the incidence of various hereditary disorders. Recent advances in genetics and medicine have shown a link between genetic factors and common diseases. The information may be utilized for the prevention of various genetic disorders through pre and post-marital genetic counseling.

To a certain extent all diseases are genetic in origin though environmental factors interfere with the expression of the genetic disorders. About 6 percent of all new born suffer from hereditary diseases and defects. It has been observed that an individual may carry about 5-8 harmful genes. The quality of life of a population is determined by these genetic as well as genetico-environmental disorders. A better quality of life could be achieved by diagnosing the genetic disorders and it's frequency in the population as well as providing genetic counseling to prevent abnormal births.

The genetic approach to quality of life and health care is an attitude. It reflects a desire to assist patients and their families in avoiding the occurrence or recurrence of the disorder. Ensuring that a family with a genetic disorder receives genetic counseling is a primary care responsibility, even though the actual genetic counseling may be carried out by a specialist in a secondary or tertiary care facility. The burdens of the disorder and its management have their greatest significance in terms of the family as a whole.

Genetic and congenital disorders are important at all levels of health care because they can involve all body parts and function and are so common. Major congenital malformations occur in 2 to 4% of all newborns up to age 14 years, congenital malformation are the third most common cause of death in both sexes. From ages 15 to 35, they are the ninth most common cause of death. Chromosome abnormalities account for at least 20% of all spontaneous abortions as well as infertility. The incidence of chromosomal aberrations among live born infants is at least 0.5%. Diseases inherited as single gene defects have a collective incidence of about 2%. Polygenic malformations such as spina bifida/ anencephaly, cleft lip/palate, club foot and congenital heart disease have individual incidence rate of about 1:1000. Other polygenic disorders, such as diabetes mellitus and hypertension are even more frequent. It has been estimated that approximately 20% of all hospital patients have a genetic contribution to their clinical problems.

The statistical detail of the genetic disorders given above throws light on the need of health care. Health care providers, by definition assume responsibility for assisting patients or families already afflicted by disease. But at all levels they must also assume responsibility for initiating measure that facilitates prevention. Because, the prevention of most of these disorders depends on a family being properly informed, emphasis must be placed on the process by which the relevant information is gathered, formulated and delivered.

CHAPTER 2

# Essentials of Genetics

## INTRODUCTION

Like most fields of study, genetics has its own language which can be used to describe any inherited trait. The Austrian monk Gregor Mendel experimented with garden pea plant for nine years. Based on his work several terms have been introduced to explain the genetic principles.

## 2.1 GENETIC TERMINOLOGY

A gene is a DNA molecule, the hereditary unit responsible for the synthesis of a protein which is required for body function. These genes are located in chromosomes the hereditary vehicle. There are 23 pairs of chromosomes in a human cell, of which a pair XX in a female and XY in a male are called sex chromosomes or **allosomes**, carry the genes that determine the sex. Non-sex determining chromosomes are termed **autosomes**. The genes carried by sex chromosomes are called sex-linked and those associated with autosomes are autosomal. Chromosomes are present in pairs, called **homologous**, one derived from the father and the other from the mother. There are 2 sets of chromosomes of 23 each, one is the paternal set and the other the maternal set. Genes for a trait is always present in pairs, called **allele**. One allele is **dominant** over the other and suppresses the expression of a **recessive** allele. A trait may be controlled by similar alleles AA / aa or dissimilar alleles Aa. The former is termed **homozygous** and the later **heterozygous**. The term **phenotype** represents the physical expression of a character and **genotype** refers to the genetic constitution of a trait. For example, considering the trait, height of a plant controlled by a pair of alleles 'A' and 'a', the phenotype may be tall and dwarf. But the genotype for tall is AA or Aa and the genotype for dwarf is aa. The normal gene which has not undergone any change is termed wild type and that has undergone change by a mutation is called mutant gene. **Mutation** is a change in the DNA molecule caused by a variety of physical, chemical and biological agents.

## 2.2 MENDEL'S LAWS IN HUMAN GENETICS

Mendel's laws of inheritance were derived from experiments with plants, but they form corner stone of the whole science of genetics. Mendel showed that information for contrasting characters segregate and recombine in simple mathematical proportions. Mendel postulated four new principles concerning unit inheritance, dominance, segregation and independent assortment that apply to most genes of all diploid organisms.

### *i Principle of Unit Inheritance*

Hereditary characters are determined by units of information which are now called as genes. An **allele** is the alternative form of a gene.

### *ii Principle of Dominance*

Alleles occur in pairs in each individual, but the effects of one allele may be masked by those of a dominant partner allele.

### *iii Law of Segregation*

During formation of the gametes the members of each pair of alleles separate, so that each gamete carries only one allele of each pair.

**Example** The ear lobes of some people have an elongated attachment to the neck, while others are free. The gene for free ear lobe is designated as 'F' and 'f' for attached ear lobe.

Consider a man carrying two copies of F (i.e. FF) for free ear lobes married to a woman with attached earlobes ff. Both can produce only one kind of gamete 'F' for the man and 'f' for the woman. All their children will have one copy of each allele Ff, and it is found that all such children have free ear lobes because F is dominant to f. The children constitute the first filial generation or F1, generation. Individuals with identical alleles are **homozygotes**; those with different alleles are **heterozygotes.**

The second filial or F2, generation is composed of the grand children of the original couple, resulting from mating of their offspring with partners of similar genotype. In each case both parents are heterozygotes, so both produce F and f gametes in equal members. This creates three genotypes in the F2: FF, Ff and ff in the genotypic ratio of 1:2:1. Due to dominance of F over f, the heterozygotes (Ff) are phenotypically similar as dominant homozygotes (FF), so there are three offsprings with free ear lobes and one with attached ear lobe. The phenotypic ratio is 3:1

**Table 2.1** Results of a cross between a man and woman heterozygous for free ear lobe (Ff)

| *Male/Female* | *F* | *f* |
|---|---|---|
| F | FF | Ff |
| f | Ff | Ff |

### *iv Law of Independent Assortment*

Different genes control different phenotypic characters and the alleles of different genes re-assort independently of one another.

**Example** 'Red' hair, occur naturally only in individuals who are homozygous for a recessive allele 'r'. Non-red is dominant, designated with the symbol R. All red-haired people are therefore 'rr' while non-red, either RR or Rr.

Consider the mating between an individual with red hair and attached ear lobes (rrff) and a partner who is heterozygous for both (RrFf). The recessive homozygote can produce only one kind of gamete, of genotype rf, but the double heterozygote can produce gametes of four genotypes; RF, Rf, rF and rf.

Off spring of four genotypes are produced: RrFf, Rrff, rrFf and rrff and these are in the ratio 1:1:1:1.

These off springs also have phenotyes that are different; non-red with free ear lobes, non-red with attached ear lobes, red with free ear lobes and red with attached ear lobes respectively.

### Matings between Double Heterozygotes

When mating between double heterozygotes happen, each can produce four kinds of gametes: RF, Rf, rF and rf, which combine at random and can produce nine different genotypic combinations. Due to dominance there are only four phenotypes in the ratio 9: 3:3:1 (total=16).

The following is the result of the above mating:—

1. A child with non-red hair and free ear lobes (RRFF, RRFf, RrFf and RrFf) as 9/16
2. A child with non-red hair and attached ear lobes (RRff, Rrff) as 3/16
3. A child with red hair and free ear lobes (rrFF, rrFf) as 3/16
4. A child with red hair and attached ear lobes (rrff) as 1/16

**Table 2.2** Results of a cross between a man and woman heterozygous for Non-red hair and free ear lobe (RrFf)

| *Male/Female* | *RF* | *Rf* | *rF* | *Rf* |
|---|---|---|---|---|
| RF | RRFF | RRFf | RrFF | RrFf |
| Rf | RRFf | RRff | RrFf | Rrff |
| rF | RrFF | RrFf | rrFF | rrFf |
| rf | RrFf | Rrff | rrFf | Rrff |

## 2.3 MENDELIAN TRAITS

In all the living organisms phenotypic characters are expressed externally but are determined by the genes residing in the chromosomes. This was first recognized by Gregor Mendel. The characters controlled by genes are termed **Mendelian traits**. These traits are often determined by a pair of genes with alternate expression.

### Kinds of Traits

The traits may be controlled by genes residing in the somatic chromosomes namely autosomes or in the sex chromosomes (XX or XY) and are called as autosomal traits or sex-linked traits respectively. Some traits are controlled by more than two alleles and are called multiple allelic traits.

Many human traits follow Mendelian inheritance predictions. Some of the human traits are listed below.

### Autosomal Traits

1. **Eye colour:** If the eyes are brown, it is due to the presence of one dominant gene. Blue, grey and green eyes are recessive trait.
2. **Tongue rolling:** The ability to curl the tongue upward from the sides is a dominant trait. The persons who can not roll the tongues possess recessive genes.
3. **Free ear lobe:** Earlobes that hang free from the ear are dominant over attached earlobes that are attached directly to the side of the head.
4. **Widow's peak:** A distinctive downward point in the hairline is known as the Widow's peak. This is a dominant trait. If the hairline is straight then recessive genes are present.
5. **Hitchiker's thumb:** The ability to bend the thumb backward (at least 45 degree) is caused by a dominant allele.
6. **Mid-digital hair:** The presence of hair on fingers is a dominant trait. Hair may not be present on all fingers, but if hair is seen even in one finger, then this is dominant phenotype.
7. **Bent little finger:** A dominant gene causes the last joint of little finger to bend inward towards the fourth finger. The straight little finger is a recessive trait.
8. **Thumb crossing:** Without thinking about it, hands are clasped together. If left thumb crosses over right then it is a dominant trait. On the other hand right over left is a recessive trait.
9. **Dimpled chin:** If dimple is noted in chin it is a dominant trait. If chin is not dimpled then it is recessive.
10. **PTC tasting:** Persons who can taste phenyl thiocarbamide bitter are termed tasters and is controlled by a dominant gene. Non-tasters do not taste it and are recessive.

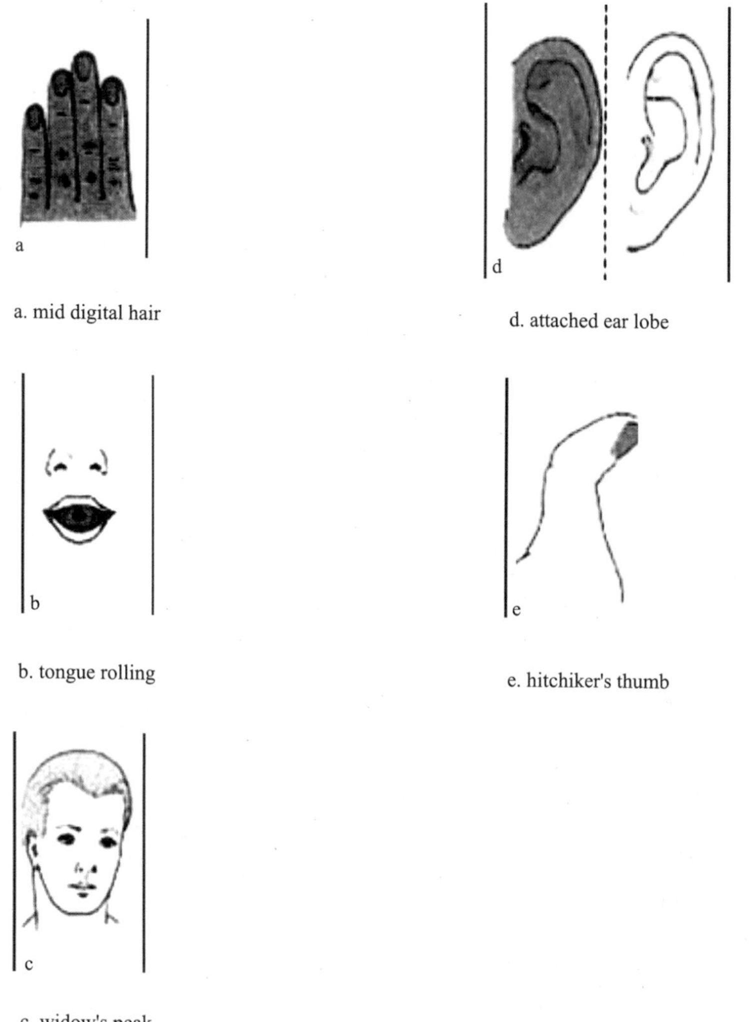


a. mid digital hair

d. attached ear lobe

b. tongue rolling

e. hitchiker's thumb

c. widow's peak

**Fig. 2.1** Mendelian traits
(Source: www.seop.yale.edu)

## 2.4 VARIATION IN GENE EXPRESSION

There are several important points to be analyzed regarding the expression of a gene which was not shown in typical Mendelian inheritance.

Though the gene responsible for a Mendelian trait controls a single phenotype, often genes tend to show many effects and are said to be pleiotropic (multiple effect). In the common example of sickle cell anemia, due to the sickle shape of the red blood cell the blood vessels become clogged. There are also other symptoms like severe physical weakness, abnormal spleen, circulatory disturbances and brain damage. Such a group of symptoms characterizing a particular condition is termed syndrome. Thus the sickle cell gene is responsible for the appearance of several changes in the normal phenotype. The term **pleiotropy** refers to the collection of effects associated with a specific gene.

The heterozygotes for sickle cell anemia carry one normal allele and another sickle cell allele ($Hb^A$ $Hb^S$ ) They are carriers. Though they are healthy they are not identical to the normal persons who carry two normal alleles ($Hb^A$ $Hb^A$). The heterozygotes are said to be sickle cell trait. This difference from the normal type is evident in blood test. In heterozygotes some cells become abnormal shaped under low oxygen tension. The terms dominant and recessive can not be applied to this pair of alleles $Hb^A$ $Hb^S$ since both kinds of hemoglobins are present. So it is evident that both alleles express themselves in the heterozygote. Such genes are said to be **codominant.** The term incomplete dominance is often used to describe conditions where the effects of one of the alleles in the heterozygotes are more pronounced than the other.

The expression of a gene may also vary from person to person. This is said to be variable expressivity. In the disease Osteogenesis imperfecta, the gene (O) responsible for the disease is dominant while its normal allele is recessive (o). In the presence of the gene O a syndrome is established. There is severe fragility of bones, weakness of ligaments and tendons, deafness and a blue coloration of the eye. However, when persons afflicted with Osteogenesis imperfecta were studied, it is shown that affected persons do not exhibit all the symptoms. For example a parent may exhibit all the symptoms while the children show only blue eye coloration. It is clear that the gene does not express itself to the same extent or in the same way in every person who carries it. A gene, whose expression is not constant and varies from one individual to the other is said to be variable expressivity.

Another feature of a gene is **penetrance.** At times, certain genes, a dominant one or a recessive one in the homozygous condition, may remain unexpressed when present in the genotype. The gene for Osteogenesis imperfecta when present it does not bring out a detectable effect in all individuals. Nine out of ten persons carrying the dominant gene will show one or more symptoms, while the remaining one will be normal. The gene has reduced penetrance. That is the gene has a penetrance of 90% expressing itself in someway. On the other hand the genes for ABO blood types are 100% penetrant that is when they are present will always be present 100%. The gene for Osteogenesis imperfecta is pleiotropic (multiple effect), shows reduced penetrance and is of variable expressivity.

The expression of any one gene may be greatly influenced by other genes present in the genotype. No genes act independently of other genes generally. The presence of one gene may completely prevent the expression of another. Eye color, for example, involves not just one pair of alleles but the interaction of many. At least three different genes have been identified which reduce the amount of melanin pigment in both skin and eyes. The third gene causes a lack of pigment only in the eye.

Certain genes, known as **modifiers,** have a slight effect on the expression of some other gene altering the expression in a quantitative way. An abnormal effect may be completely suppressed by the presence of some other gene. Such gene which prevents the expression of some other gene is termed **suppressor**.

Interaction of genes is also influenced by environment. An individual whose phenotype has been environmentally altered so that it mimics the phenotype usually related to genotype is called **phenocopy**. The familiar example is that caused by the drug thalidomide, an ingredient in certain sleeping pills. The thalidomide tragedy became evident in Europe with an increase in the birth of babies without limbs called **phocomelia** following the consumption of this drug by pregnant women. The victims phenotypically resemble those individuals who have reduced limbs due to a rare hereditary disorder produced by a dominant gene. However the thalidomide victims possess a normal genotype for limb development. Though they are limbless these individuals will transmit only the normal genes. In the study of human genetics gene interactions must be considered and the influence of environment in gene expression is never to be ignored.

## 2.5 MULTIPLE ALLELES

Multiple alleles can be defined as a set of three, four or more alleles or allelomorphic genes, which have arisen as a result of mutation of a normal gene and which occupy the same locus in the homologous chromosomes.

### Characteristics of Multiple Alleles

1. Multiple alleles occupy the same locus within the homologous chromosomes. It means only one member of the series present in a given chromosome.
2. Since in a diploid cell only two chromosomes of each type are present, only two genes of the multiple series are found in an individual.
3. Crossing over does
4. Multiple alleles co
5. In the multiple alle ... ome times they are codominant.

**Example** The ABO bloo ... es. Blood from an individual cannot always b ... the fact that blood proteins of one individual di ... tances in the blood known as **antigens** or **aggl** ... gens **A** and **B** are located in the RBC and the ... ntigen A then the antibody b is present in th ... saccharides. The clumping reaction occurs be ... **gglutination**.

Depending upon the pr ... roups have been differentiated. These are des ... ons belonging to blood group A have antigen- ... in their plasma. Persons of blood group B hav ... tibody a (anti A) in the plasma. Persons of grou ... antibodies in the plasma. Persons of group O ha ... ntibodies in their plasma. The following table r ... different blood groups.

Table 2.3 Distribution of antigens and antibodies in blood groups

| *Blood Groups* | *Antigens in RBC* | *Antibodies in plasma* |
|---|---|---|
| A | A | b (anti-B) |
| B | B | a (anti-A) |
| AB | A and B | NO |
| O | NO | a and b |

The agglutination reaction has significance in blood transfusion. The persons with blood group O lack antigens and their blood is not clumped by the serum of any blood group, so that person of O group can give blood to all but can receive blood only from O blood group. Hence these are called **universal donors**. The serum from AB blood group individuals does not cause clumping with any group. Hence they can take blood from the persons of any blood groups but can receive blood only from AB blood group persons only. So they are known as **universal recipients**.

Table 2.4 Possible effects of transfusion of blood

| *Donor's group* | *Can give to* | *Can receive from* | *Remark* |
|---|---|---|---|
| O | O, A, B, AB | O | Universal Donor |
| A | A & AB | O, A | - |
| B | B & AB | O, B | - |
| AB | AB | O, A, B, AB | Universal recipient |

## Inheritance of ABO Blood Groups

Bernstein discovered that the inheritance of ABO blood groups is by multiple alleles, $I^A$, $I^B$, i. The $I^A$ and $I^B$ genes are **codominant** and so are equally expressed. On the otherhand the i gene is recessive to both the genes $I^A$ and $I^B$.

Table 2.5 The genotypes of the blood groups

| *Blood Group* | *Genotypes* |
|---|---|
| A | $I^A I^A$ or $I^A i$ |
| B | $I^B I^B$ or $I^B i$ |
| AB | $I^A I^B$ |
| O | i i |

If the parent blood groups are known the blood groups of their children can be predicted. The following table gives the possible blood group combination in parent and the possible blood group in the offspring.

**Table 2.6** Blood groups of parents and the possible types in children

| *Parents blood group* | *Blood group in offspring* |
|---|---|
| O x O | O |
| O x A | A, O |
| O x B | B, O |
| O x AB | A, B |
| A x A | A, O |
| A x B | A, B, AB, O |
| A x AB | A, B, AB |
| B x B | B, O |
| B x AB | A, B, AB |
| AB x AB | A, B, AB |

The blood group A has been divided into subgroups $\mathbf{A_1}$, $\mathbf{A_2}$, $\mathbf{A_3}$ and $\mathbf{A_4}$ depending on the presence of specific antigens and its reaction with B-serum. The $A_1$ is common. Each of the sub groups of A is determined by a separate gene and all these genes are alleles. The genes $A_2$, $A_3$, and $A_4$, usually occur in combination with $A_1$ and $A_1$ is dominant over all the other A subtypes.

In a person of blood group AB, there might be many of these subtypes present and therefore AB blood group can be divided into subgroups $A_1B$, $A_2B$, $A_3B$, and $A_4B$.

## MN Blood Groups

Landsteiner and Levine discovered antigens M and N in human blood, which when injected into rabbits stimulated antibody production in rabbits. Human population can be divided into blood group **M,** blood group **N** or blood group **MN** depending on the presence of antigens M, N and MN respectively, but their serum does not contain antibodies.

MN blood groups are controlled by alleles M and N which are equally dominant and so they are codominant.

## Rh Factor

The Rh factor in the blood was first observed by Landsteiner and Wiener in the Rhesus monkey ***Macaca rhesus***. The red cells of the monkeys contain the antigen Rh. In human it was found out that some persons possess antigen Rh and others do not have it. Those with antigens are termed **Rh positive** and those who do not have it as **Rh negative**. According to Fischer there are three dominant genes **CDE** determining the Rh positive blood group and recessive alleles, **cde** determining Rh negative blood group. If the alleles are cde then the blood group is Rh negative. On the other hand Rh positive blood group is determined by the following combinations, Cde, CDe, CdE, CDE, cDE, CDe and cdE.

The Rh factor has great significance in child birth. The **Rh incompatibilities** and the disease caused namely **Erythroblastosis fetalis** is discussed in chapter 10.12.

## 2.6 POLYGENIC INHERITANCE

The majority of genetic traits exhibit minimum two contrasting phenotypes. Such traits are designated as qualitative or discontinuous traits. For example in garden pea plants the seed is either yellow or green and the plants are either tall or dwarf; in cattle, they may have horns or no horns; human may have blood group A or B or AB or O ; Drosophila may have red eyes or white eyes.

But there are traits where a gradation in the trait is observed. For example if a group of persons is classified according to their heights, a gradual gradation in the height can be easily noted. Such traits exhibit continuous phenotypic variation. F.C. Galton (1883) noted that many of these continuous variations are observed in human beings and are inherited. Characters like height, weight, skin color or intelligence exhibit gradual differences. These characters are often determined by a number of genes and all of them have cumulative or additive effect. Each gene contributes a certain amount of effect. The degree of expression of a trait then depends upon the number of genes present. If the number of dominant genes are more, then the degree of expression of the character will be more. This kind of inheritance is termed as **quantitative inheritance** or **polygenic inheritance**. The genes involved in this kind of inheritance are known as polygenes. So polygenes are defined as, two or more different pairs of genes which are non-allelic, having cumulative effect and are responsible for quantitative characters.

### Characteristics of Polygenes

1. The effects of each contributing gene are cumulative or additive.
2. Each contributing gene produces an equal effect.
3. There is no dominance involved.
4. The polygenes have pleiotropic effects, that is, one gene may modify or suppress more than one phenotypic trait. A single gene may do only one thing chemically but may affect many characters.
5. The environmental conditions have considerable effect on the phenotypic expression of polygenes. In plants for example the height may be attend by soil, water, temperature, light or nutrition. Similarly identical twins with similar genotypes, if grow up in different environments, show different IQ. The skin color of one person can be lighter or darker depending upon the amount of exposure to sunlight.

**Examples**

### Skin Color in Man

A classical example of polygenic inheritance was given by Davenport (1913) in Jamaica. The presence of melanin pigment in the skin determines the skin color. The more is the pigment the darker is the skin color. The amount of melanin developing in an individual is determined by two pairs of genes. There genes are present at two different loci and each dominant gene is responsible for the synthesis of fixed amount of melanin. The effect of all the genes is additive and the amount of melanin produced is always proportional to the number of dominant genes. Davenport found that the two pairs of genes A – a and B – b cause the difference in skin pigmentation between Negro and

Caucasian population. A Negro, has four dominant genes AABB, and a Caucasian has four recessive genes aabb. The $F_1$ offspring of mating of aabb with AABB, are all AaBb and have an intermediate skin colour termed **mulatto**. A mating of two such mulatoes produces a wide variety of skin colour in the offspring, ranging from skins as dark as the original Negro parent to as white as the original Caucasian parents. The results of this cross are as follows:

**Table 2.7** Inheritance of skin color in man

| | | Negro AABB | X | White aabb | $P_1$ |
|---|---|---|---|---|---|
| AaBb | X | Mulatto AaBb | | Mulatto $F_1$ | |

| ♀ ♂ | *AB* | *Ab* | *aB* | *ab* |
|---|---|---|---|---|
| AB | AABB | AABb | ABBa | ABab |
| Ab | AABb | AAbb | AaBb | Aabb |
| aB | AaBB | AaBb | AaBB | ABab |
| ab | AaBb | Aabb | abaB | Abab |

**$F_2$ results**

| Phenotypes | Genotypes | Genotypic frequency ratio | Phenotypic |
|---|---|---|---|
| Black (Negro) | AABB | 1 | 1 |
| Dark | AaBB | 2 | 4 |
| | AABb | 2 | |
| Intermediate | AaBb | 4 | |
| (Mulalto) | aaBB | 1 | 6 |
| | AAbb | 1 | |
| Light | Aabb | 2 | 4 |
| | aaBb | 2 | |
| White | aabb | 1 | 1 |

These results clearly indicate that a and B, the dominant genes produce about the same amount of skin pigmentation. Therefore the decrease or increase in number of A and B genes cause different phenotypes. There is graduation in skin phenotypes as black (4 dominant genes), dark (3 dominant genes), mulatto (2 dominant genes), light (1 dominant gene) and white (O dominant genes). The phenotypic ratio is 1 black : 4 dark : 6 mulatto : 4 light : 1 white.

## Height in Man

Skin color in man is a simple example of polygenic inheritance since only 2 pairs of genes are involved. But the inheritance of height in man is more complex as there are ten or more pairs of genes involved in controlling the trait. In man the tallness is recessive to shortness. So an individual having the genotype of more dominant genes will have shortness as their phenotype. This polygenic trait is controlled by a multiple pairs of genes and is variously influenced by a variety of environmental conditions. The heights of adults generally range from 140 cm to 203 cm. If the height of a thousand adult men is measured and the individual height is plotted against height in centimeters and the points connected, a bell shaped curve is produced and is termed normal distribution curve and is characteristic of quantitative inheritance.

CHAPTER 3

# Chromosomal basis of Heredity

## INTRODUCTION

In the 1870s, the importance of nucleus and its contents was recognized by the observation that the nuclei of two gametes fuse in the process of fertilization. The next major advance was the discovery of chromosomes, which became visible by light microscopy when stained with basic dyes. Then, chromosomes were found to segregate by an orderly process into daughter cells in cell division.

Each species of plant and animal has a characteristic number of chromosomes per cell. For example fruit flies have 8 and human 46. There is no significance between the complexity of an organism and its number of chromosomes.

Generally there are two sets of chromosomes. This is the consequence of sexual reproduction; one set inherited from the father and another from the mother. Each chromosome in one set has a corresponding chromosome in the other set, together constituting a homologous pair. Human cells for example, have 46 chromosomes, comprising 23 homologous pairs. The two chromosomes of a homologous pair is similar in structure and size, and each carries genetic information for the same set of heredity characteristics. A trait is often represented by a pair of alleles (the alternative forms of a gene) residing in the homologous pair. Thus most cells carry two sets of genetic information and these cells are **diploid.** In contrast the reproductive cells have only one set of chromosomes and are **haploid**.

## 3.1 CHROMOSOME STRUCTURE

Chromosomes are visible only when the cell is undergoing division. Each chromosome has a single molecule of DNA which is highly folded and condensed. A functional chromosome has three elements: a centromere, a pair of telomeres and origins of replication.

The **centromere** is the attachment point for spindle fibers aiding chromosome movement during cell division. On the basis of centromere location chromosomes were classified into four types. In **metacentric** chromosome the centromere is in the mid point thereby dividing the chromosome into two equal halves. If the centromere is away from the mid point, a long arm (q arm) and a short arm (p arm) can be distinguished and the chromosme is termed **submetacentric**. In **telocentric** chromosomes the centromere is at the end of the chromosome that there is only one arm. If the centromere is at the extreme end of the chromosome then it is termed **acrocentric**.

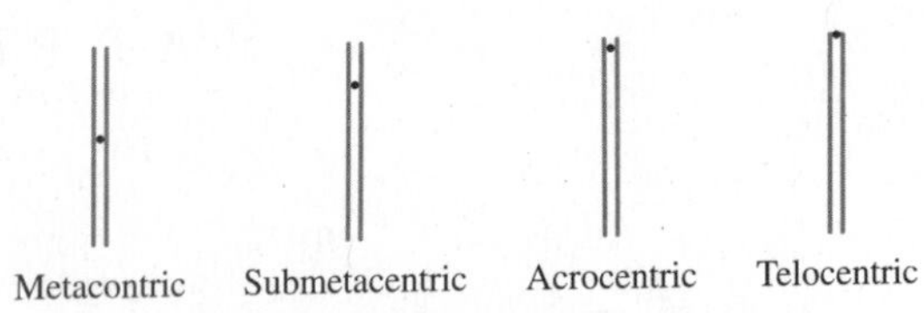


**Fig. 3.1** Chromosome types

**Telomeres** are the natural ends (the tips) of a linear chromosome. They provide chromosome stability.

Origins of replication are the sites where DNA synthesis begins. Each chromosome replicates in cell division to make a copy of itself. These identical copies, called **sister chromatids** are held together at centromere. Each sister chromatid consists of a single molecule of DNA.

The eukaryotic DNA is closely associated with proteins to form structures called **chromatin**. The two basic types of chromatin are: **euchromatin**, which undergoes changes in cell cycle, and **heterochromatin**, which remains in a highly condensed state throughout cell cycle. Euchromatin constitutes the majority of the chromosomal material, while heterochromatin is present in specific places like centromere and telomere.

The most abundant proteins in chromatin are the **histones**, and are of five types: H1, H2A, H2B, H3 and H4. All these proteins give a net positive charge. The positive charge attracts the negative charge on the phosphates of DNA and holds the DNA in contact with the histones. There are also **nonhistone chromosomal proteins** constituting major part of the chromosomal material. The **chromosomal scaffold proteins** play a role in folding and packing of the chromosome. The nonhistone proteins are components (enzymes) of replication and transcription.

Under electron microscope the chromatin appears to be a beaded structure. The bead like units in the chromatin is called **nucleosome**. It has a core particle consisting of DNA wrapped about two times around an octamer of eight histone proteins like a thread around a spool. The H1 protein sits inside the coils of the nucleosome. It helps to lock the DNA into place, acting as a clamp around the nucleosome octamer. Together, the core particle and its associated H1 proteins are called the **chromatosome**. These are located at regular intervals along the DNA molecule and are separated from one another by **linker DNA** and most cells have about 30bp to 40bp of linker DNA.

## 3.2 CELL DIVISION

The stages through which a cell pass from one stage to the other is called **cell cycle.** It is significant in that the genetic information is passed from parent to daughter cells through cell cycle. The cell

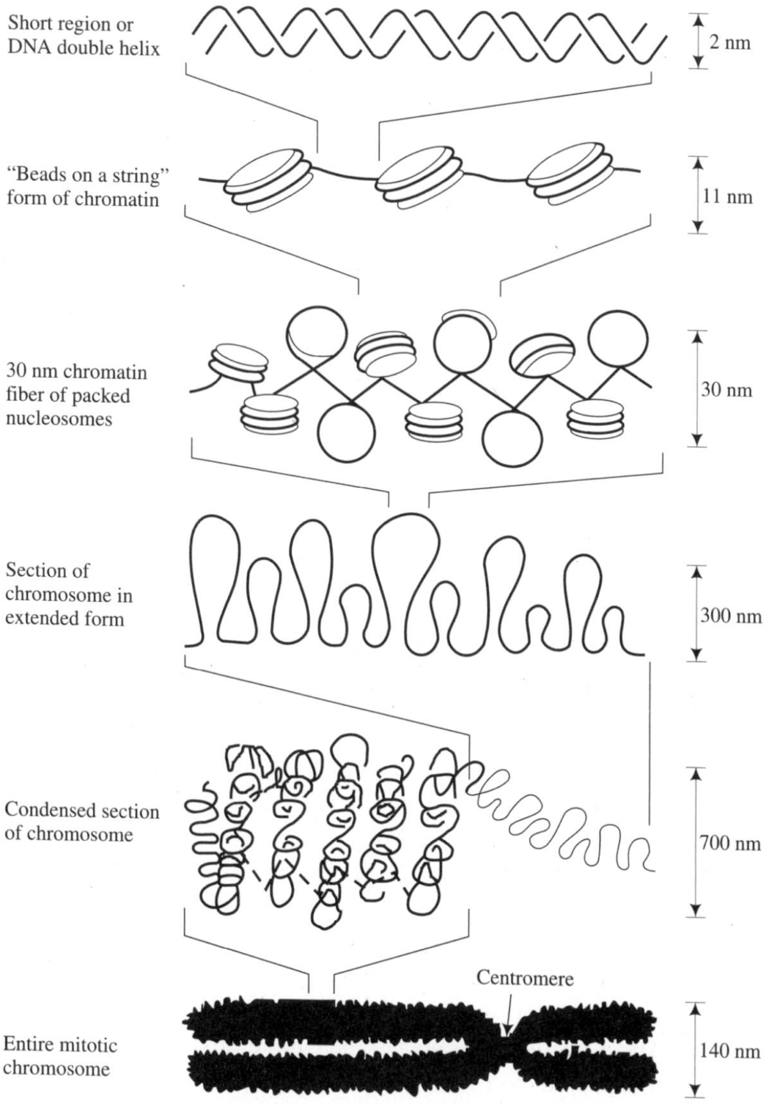


**Fig. 3.2** Chromosome fine structure (Source: www.home.planet.nl)

cycle consists of two major phases. The first is **interphase**, the period between cell divisions, in which the cell grows and matures. The second is **M phase** (mitotic phase), the period of active cell division. M phase includes nuclear division namely **mitosis** and cytoplasmic division namely **cytokinesis**.

Interphase is divided into three phases: $G_1$, S and $G_2$. Interphase begins with $G_1$ (gap 1) where cell grows and proteins are synthesized. There is a critical point in the cell cycle, termed the **$G_1$ /S checkpoint**, in $G_1$; after this check point has been passed, the cell divides. Before reaching the $G_1$ /

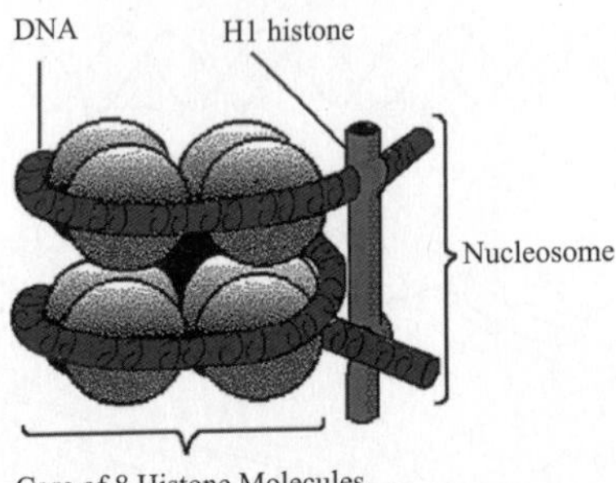


**Fig. 3.3** Nucleosome structure
(Source: accessexcellence.org)

S checkpoint, cells may exit from the active cell cycle and enter into a non dividing phase called $G_0$, a stable state in which cells maintain a constant size.

After $G_1$, the cell enters the S phase (DNA synthesis), in which the chromosome duplicates. If DNA synthesis is blocked, the cell will not be able to undergo mitosis. Following S phase each chromosome contains two chromatids.

After the S phase, the cell enters $G_2$ (gap 2). In this phase, several biochemical events necessary for cell division take place. The important **$G_2$/M checkpoint** is reached in $G_2$: after this checkpoint, the cell is ready to divide and enters M phase. The time duration of Interphase varies from cell to cell. A typical mammalian cell spends about 10 hours in $G_1$, 9 hours in S, and 4 hours in $G_2$.

M phase is the part of the cell cycle in which the chromatids are separated and the cell undergoes division. The resulting cells receive complete set of genetic information. M phase is usually divided into six stages: prophase, prometaphase, metaphase, anaphase and telophase (mitotic stages) and cytokinesis.

Chromosomes condense during **prophase**. Each chromosome possesses two chromatids. The mitotic spindle that moves the chromosomes is formed. The spindle grows out from a pair of **centrosomes** that migrates to opposite sides of the cell. Within each centrosome is a **centriole** which is also made of microtubules.

**Prometaphase** is marked by the disintegration of nuclear membrane. Spindle microtubules enter the nuclear region. These microtubules anchor the chromatids to both of the centrosomes. The microtubules pull the chromosomes.

During **metaphase,** the chromosomes arrange in a single plane, the metaphase plate between the two centrosomes. The centrosomes are now at the opposite ends of the cell with microtubule radiating outward and meeting in the middle of the cell.

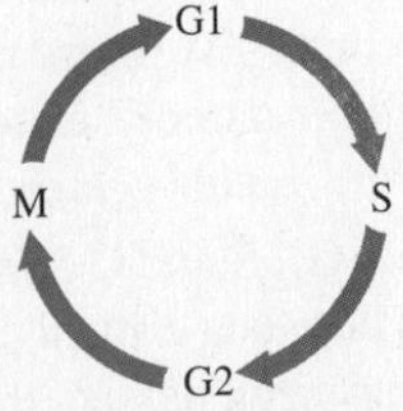


**Fig. 3.4** Cell cycle

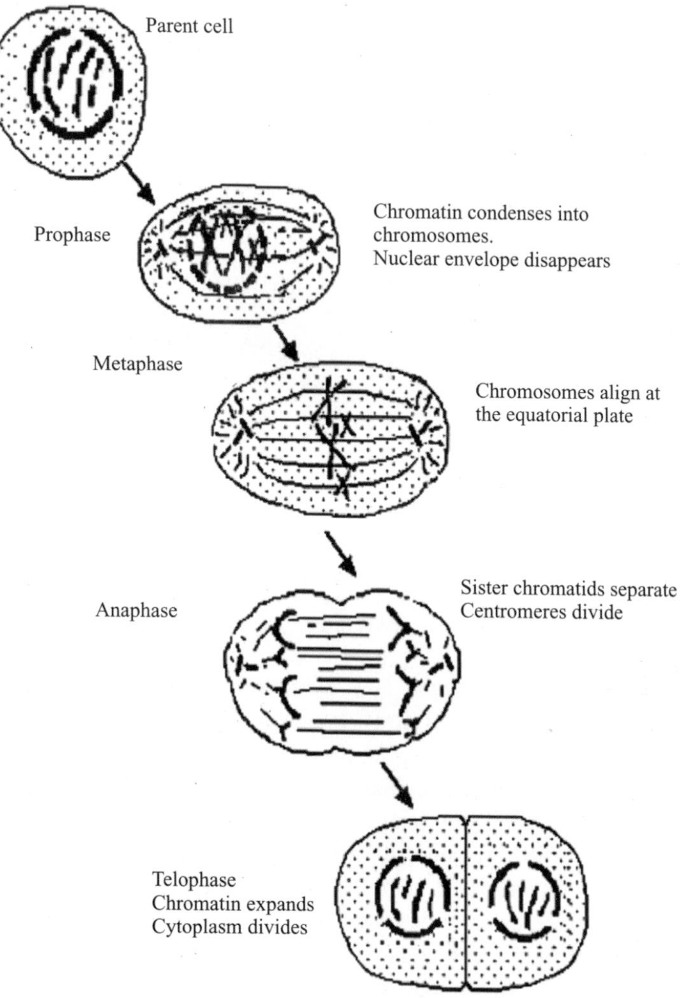


**Fig. 3.5** Stages of Mitosis
(Source: www.biology.iupui.edu)

**Anaphase** begins when the sister chromatids separate and move toward opposite poles. After the chromatids are separated they are considered as a separate chromosome.

**Telophase** is marked by the arrival of the chromosomes at the poles. The nuclear membrane is formed around the chromosome and produce two nuclei. There is simultaneous division of cytoplasm namely **cytokinesis** resulting in two daughter cells.

In reproductive cells the cell division is termed **Meiosis** which leads to gamete formation where the chromosome number is reduced to half. This is significant because in fertilization the two haploid gametes fuse to produce a diploid zygote. Meiosis consists of two phases: meiosis I and meiosis II each including a cell division. The first division is a reduction division where the actual number of chromosome is reduced to half. The second division is similar to mitosis.

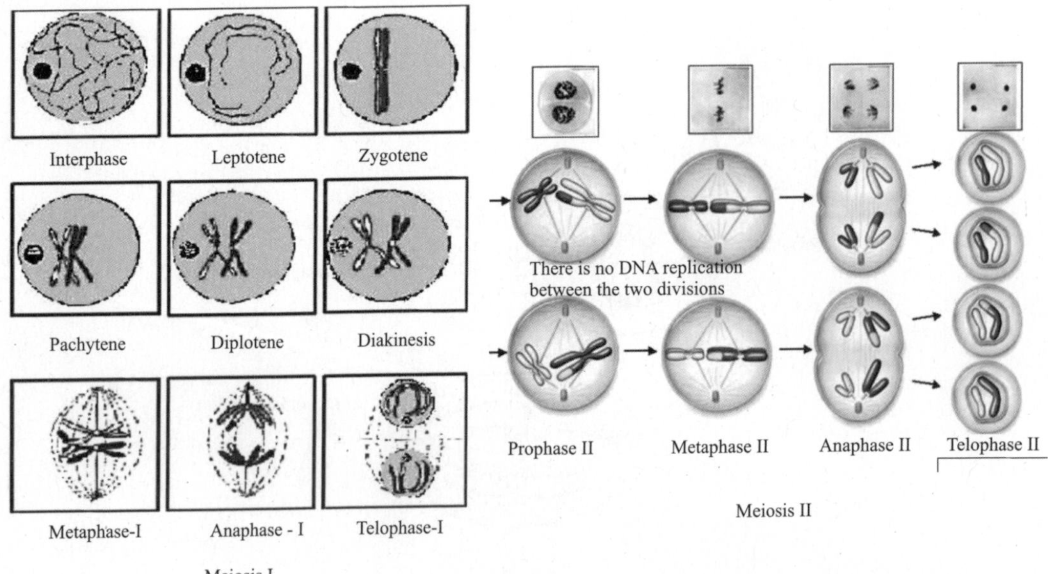


**Fig. 3.6** Stages of Meiosis
(Source: www.biology.iupui.edu)

**Meiosis I** consists of the following events. **Prophase I** is a long one and divided into five stages. In **leptotene**, the chromosomes contract and become visible. In **zygotene**, the homologous chromosomes pair and begin **synapsis**, a close pairing of chromosomes. Each synapsed chromosome consists of four chromatids called a bivalent or tetrad. In **pachytene** the chromosomes become shorter and thicker. Crossing over and exchange of genetic material takes place. In **diplotene** the centromeres of the paired chromosomes move apart and the homologous chromosomes remain attached at point called **chiasma** which is the result of crossing over. In **diakinesis** chromosome condensation continues and the chiasmata move towards the tips and so the chromosomes remain paired at the ends of the chromosomes only. At the end of prophase I, nuclear membrane breaks down and spindle forms.

**Metaphase I** begin when homologous pairs of chromosomes align at the equatorial plane. A microtubule from one pole attaches to one chromosome of a homologous pair and a microtubule from the other pole attaches to the other chromosome of the pair. In **Anaphase I** the homologous chromosomes separate. They are pulled towards opposite poles. The sister chromatids remain attached and move together. In **Telophase** I, the chromosomes arrive at the poles and the cytoplasm divides.

**Interkinesis** is the period between Meiosis I and Meiosis II. Here the nuclear membrane is formed around the chromosomes. These cells then undergo **Prophase II.** In this stage the events are reversed. The chromosomes re-condens, the spindle is re-formed and the nuclear membrane once again breaks up. **Metaphase II** is similar to metaphase of mitosis. The chromosomes occupy the metaphase plate and the sister chromatids face opposite poles. In **Anaphase II**, the sister chromatids separate and the chromatids are pulled to opposite poles. Each chromatid now becomes a separate chromosome. In **Telophase II**, The chromosomes arrive at the poles, a nuclear membrane is re-formed around the chromosomes and the cytoplasm divides.

## Control of the Cell Cycle

Cell cycle is highly regulated. There is an internal clock for every cell regarding the maximum number times that it can divide in a culture. It is called **Hayflick limit**. A connective tissue cell from a fetus, for example, divides in culture from 35 to 63 times. However a similar cell from an adult divides only 14 to 29 times. Within an organism, different cell types undergo mitosis at different rates. The cells of the intestinal epithelium divide throughout life; a cell in the brain may never divide; a cell in the deepest skin layer of a 90 year could divide more times if the person lives longer.

Factors from outside can stimulate cell division. These include **hormones** and **growth factors**. Cells are also influenced by proteins within them. Groups of proteins called **kinases** and **cyclins** activate the genes and whose products carry out mitosis. The biochemical named **maturation promoting factor** (MPF) stimulates cell division. MPF is a two protein complex. One protein is a regulator protein, called cdc2 kinase which controls the cell cycle in all the organisms. Cdc2 kinase binds to another protein called cyclin, which has accumulated during the previos interphase, forming a pre-MPF molecule. An enzyme activates pre-MPF to become mature MPF. The presence of this stimulates mitosis. MPF also stimulates enzymes that break down cyclin, stopping MPF's activity. With no active, levels of cyclin-degrading enzyme decrease and cyclin accumulates again. When cyclin combines with kinase which is always present, division begins again. Any abnormality in cell cycle results in cancer and other growth disorder.

CHAPTER 4

# The Genetic Material

## INTRODUCTION

The unit of heredity is termed gene. Genes are segments of DNA. Chromosomes contain DNA which is the genetic material. They are transmited from parent cell to daughter cells during mitosis. Following meiosis and fusion of male and female gametes they are passed on from one generation to the other. DNA plays an important role in all the activities of an organism.

## 4.1 HISTORY

DNA was first isolated by Friedrich Miescher who, in 1869, discovered a microscopic substance in the pus of discarded surgical bandage. As it resided in the nuclei of cells, he called it 'nuclein'. In 1929 Levene suggested that DNA consisted of a string of nucleotide units. In 1937 William Astbury produced the first X-ray diffraction patterns that showed that DNA has regular structure.

In 1943 Oswald Theodore Avery discovered that in ***Pneumococcus***, one type can be transformed to another type by the 'transforming principle' namely DNA. DNA's role in heredity was confirmed by Alfred Hershey and Martha Chase in 1953, in the Hershy-Chase experiment which showed that DNA is the genetic material of the T2 phage.

In 1953 based on X-ray diffraction images by Rosalind Franklin and the information that the bases are paired, James D. Watson and Francis Crick suggested the accepted double helix model of DNA.

In 1957 Crick laid out the 'Central Dogma' of molecular biology, which explains the relationship between DNA, RNA and proteins. The DNA replication mechanism proved by

Meselson and Stahl experiment in 1958 supported double helical structure of DNA. Further work by Crick and coworkers showed that genetic code was based on triplets of bases, called codons, allowing Har Gobind Khorana and Marshall Warren Nirenberg to decipher the genetic code. These findings represent the birth of molecular biology.

## 4.2 DNA

Deoxyribonucleic acid (DNA) is a nucleic acid that contains the genetic information for the development and functioning of living organisms. All living things contain DNA genomes. A possible exception is a group of viruses that have RNA genomes. The main role of DNA in the cell is the long-term storage of information. The genome is often compared to a set of blueprints, since it contains the instructions to construct other components of the cell, such as proteins and RNA molecules. The DNA segments that carry this genetic information are called genes, but other DNA sequences have structural purposes, or are involved in regulating the expression of genetic information.

In eukaryotes DNA is stored inside the cell nucleus, while in prokaryotes the DNA is in the cell cytoplasm. Unlike enzymes, DNA does not participate directly in most of the biochemical reactions it controls; rather, various enzymes act on DNA and copy its information into either more DNA, in DNA replication or transcribe and translate into protein. In chromosomes, chromatin proteins such as histones compact and organize DNA, which helps controlling the interactions with other proteins in the nucleus.

The major function of DNA is to encode the sequence of amino acid residues in proteins, using the genetic code. To read the genetic code, cells make a copy of a stretch of DNA in the Ribonucleic acid (RNA). Some RNA copies are used to direct protein biosynthesis, but others are used directly as parts of ribosomes.

### Chemical Structure of DNA

DNA is a long **polymer** made from repeating units called **nucleotides**. The DNA chain is 22 to 24 A° and one nucleotide unit is 3.3 A° long. Although these repeating units are very small, DNA polymers can be enormous molecules containing millions of nucleotides. For example, the largest human chromosome, chromosome number 1, is 220 million base pairs long. DNA is made of two long strands entwine to form a double helix. The nucleotide repeats contain both the backbone of the molecule, which holds the chain together, and a base, which interacts with the other DNA strand in the helix. In general, a base linked to a sugar is called a **nucleoside** and a base linked to a sugar and one or more phosphate group is called a nucleotide. If multiple nucleotides are linked together, as in DNA, this polymer is referred to as a polynucleotide.

The backbone of the DNA is made from alternating phosphate and sugar residues. The sugar in DNA is the pentose (five carbon) sugar 2-deoxyribose. The sugars are joined together by phosphate groups that form phosphodiester bonds between the third and fifth carbon atoms of adjacent sugar rings. In a double helix the direction of the nucleotides in one strand is opposite to their direction in the other strand. This arrangement of DNA strands is called antiparallel. The asymmetric ends of a strand of DNA bases are referred to as the 5' (five prime) and 3' (three prime) ends. One of the major differences between DNA and RNA is the sugar, with 2-deoxyribose being replaced by the alternative pentose sugar ribose in RNA.

The DNA double helix is stabilized by the hydrogen bonds between the bases attached to the two strands. The four bases found in DNA are **adenine** (A), **cytosine** (C), **guanine** (G) and **thymine** (T). These four bases are attached to the sugar/phosphate to form the complete nucleotide.

These bases are classified into two types; adenine and guanine are fused five and six-membered hetercyclic compounds called **purines**, while cytosine and thymine are six-membered rings called **pyrimidines**. A fifth pyrimidine base called uracil (U), usually replaces thymine in RNA and differs from thymine by lacking a methyl group on its ring.

The helix is a right-handed spiral. As the DNA strands wind around each other, they leave gaps between each set of phosphate backbones, revealing the sides of the bases inside. There are two of these grooves twisting around the surface of the double helix: one groove is 22 A° wide and the other is 12 A° wide. The larger groove is called major groove, while the smaller, narrower groove is called minor groove. The narrowness of the minor groove means that the edges of the bases are more accessible in the major groove. As a result, proteins like transcription factors that can bind to specific sequences in double-stranded DNA usually read the sequence by making contacts to the sides of the bases exposed in the major groove.

## Base Pairing

Each type of base on one strand forms a bond with just one type of base on the other strand. This is called complementary base pairing. Purines form hydrogen bonds to pyrimidines, with A bonding only to T, and C bonding only to G. This arrangement of two nucleotides joined across the double helix is called a base pair. In a double helix, the two strands are also held together by hydrophobic forces. As hydrogen bonds are not covalent, they can be broken and rejoined relatively easy. The two strands of DNA in a double helix can therefore be pulled apart like a zipper, either by a mechanical force or high temperature. As a result of this complementarity, all the information in the double stranded sequence of a DNA helix is duplicated on each strand, which is vital in DNA replication. This reversible and specific interaction between complementary base pairs is critical for all the functions of DNA.

The two types of base pairs form different numbers of hydrogen bonds, AT forming two hydrogen bonds, and GC forming three hydrogen bonds. The GC base pair is therefore stronger than the AT base pair.

## Supercoiling

DNA can be twisted like a rope in a process called DNA supercoiling. Normally, with DNA in its 'relaxed' state, a strand circles the axis of the double helix once every 10.4 base pairs, but if the DNA is twisted the strands become more tightly or more loosely wound. If the DNA is twisted in the direction of the helix, this is positive supercoiling**,** and the bases are held more tight together. If they are twisted in the opposite direction, this is negative supercoiling, and the bases come apart more easily.

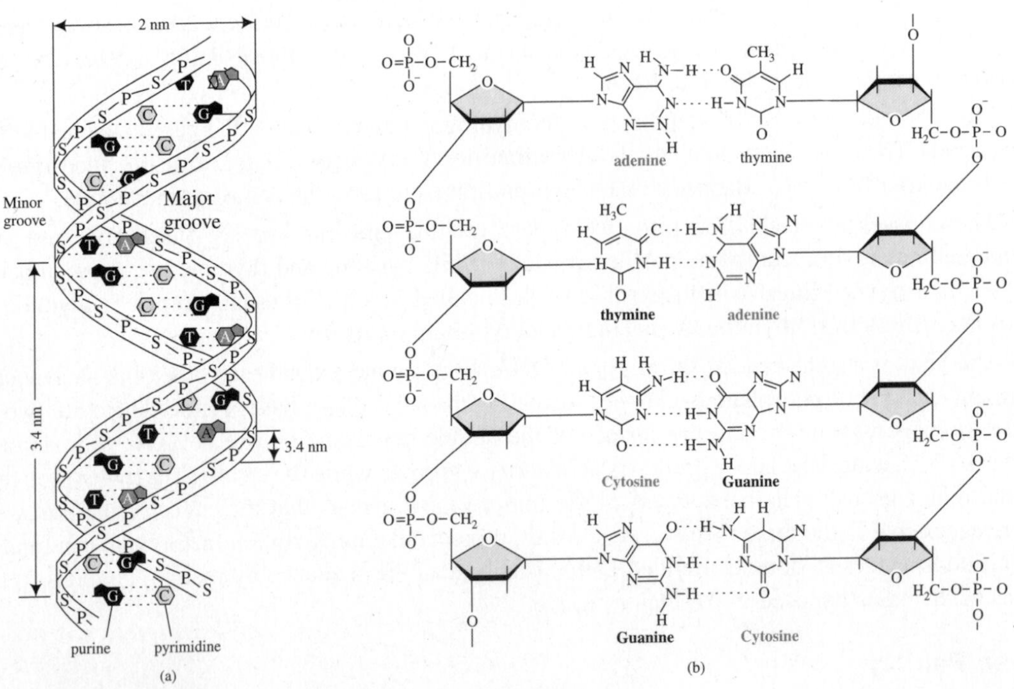


**Fig. 4.1** Structure of DNA
(Source: www.academic.brooklyn.cuny.edu)

## Alternative Structures

DNA exists in several possible conformations. The conformations so far identified are: A-DNA, B-DNA, C-DNA, D-DNA, E-DNA, H-DNA, L-DNA and Z-DNA. However only A-DNA, B-DNA and Z-DNA are believed to be found in nature. The DNA conformation depends on the sequence of the DNA, the amount and direction of supercoiling, chemical modifications of the bases and also solution conditions, such as the concentration of metal ions and polyamines. Of these three conformations, the **B form** is most common.

The **A form** is wider right-handed spiral, with a shallow and wide minor groove and a narrower and deeper major groove. Segments of DNA where the bases have been methylated may undergo a larger change in conformation and adopt the **Z form**. Here, the strands turn about the helical axis in a left-handed spiral, the opposite of the more common B form.

## Quadruplex Structures

At the ends of the linear chromosomes are specialized regions of DNA called telomeres. In human cells, telomeres are usually lengths of single stranded DNA containing several thousands of repeats of a simple TTAGGG sequence. These guanine-rich sequences may stabilize chromosome ends by forming very unusual quadruplex structures. Here, four guanine bases form a flat plate, through hydrogen bonding, and these flat four-base units then stack on top of each other, to form a stable quadruplex. The single DNA strand forms a loop, with the sets of four bases stacking in a central quadruplex three pates deep. In the space at the centre of the stacked base are three chelated potassium ions. Other structures can also be formed and the central set of four bases can come from either one folded strand, or several different parallel strands.

Telomeres often form large loops. These are called telomere loops or **T-loop**. Here, the single stranded DNA curls around in a circle, stabilized by telomere-binding proteins. The very end of the T-loop, the single-stranded telomere DNA is held onto a region of double-stranded DNA by the telomere strand disrupting the double-helical DNA and base pairing to one of the two strands. This triple-stranded structure is called a displacement loop or **D-loop**.

## Sense and Antisense

A DNA sequence is called **'sense'** if its sequence is the same as that of a messenger RNA (mRNA) copy that is translated into protein. The sequence on the opposite strand is complementary to the sense sequence and is therefore called **'antisense'** sequence. Both sense and antisense sequences can exist on different parts of the same strand of DNA.

## Mitochondrial DNA

DNA occurs in the nucleus and it forms the major part of the chromosomes. In the cytoplasm, DNA occurs in the mitochondria in small amount. The mitochondrial DNA (mDNA) differs from the nuclear DNA in that the DNA strand is joined at the end to form a ring and the composition of nitrogenous bases also differ. In a zygote the mitochondria is wholly derived from the ovum. So the mitochondrial genes show strictly **maternal inheritance**.

## Biological Functions

The genetic information carried by DNA, responsible for a trait is termed gene. Genetic information in genes is transmitted through complementary base pairing. When a cell uses the information in a gene, the DNA sequence is copied into a complementary RNA sequence in a process called transcription. This RNA copy is then used to make a matching protein sequence in a process called **translation**. Alternatively, a cell may copy its genetic information in a process called DNA **replication**.

## DNA Replication

Cell division is essential for an organism to grow, but when cell divides it must also replicate the DNA so that the two daughter cells have the same genetic information as their parent. The double stranded DNA provides simple mechanism for DNA replication. Replication occurs by separation of the two strands, with each single strand serving as a **template** for a new strand. The nucleotides are strung together one after another opposite the template strand thus resulting in two identical stands. **DNA polymerase** enzyme is responsible for replication which travels along the old DNA strand and aids in bonding of new nucleotides.

In eukaryotes DNA replicates at many sites at the same time. The two strands are untwisted at many places and the bases are exposed for enzyme binding and complementary nucleotide attachment. Each local separation appears to be a bubble.

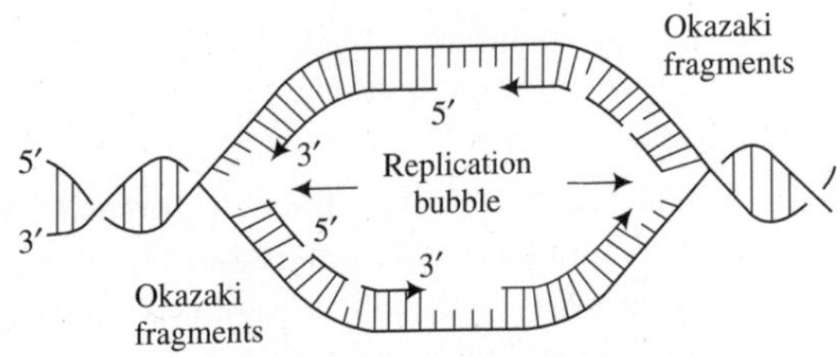


**Fig. 4.2** DNA replication
(Source: www.geneticengineering.org)

The two strands of the original double helix run in opposite directions and so the two new strands forming at one of the ends of a replicating bubble cannot be synthesized in the same direction. For example if the Y- shaped replication fork at the right side of the bubble is considered the upper branch of the replication fork can add nucleotides at 3' end but the lower branch proceed backward. The new fragments thus formed are called **Okazaki fragments**. These fragments are joined together by the enzyme **DNA ligase**.

### Genetic Code

Within a gene, the sequence of bases along a DNA strand defines a messenger RNA sequence, which then defines a protein sequence. The relationship between the nucleotide sequences of genes and the amino acid sequences of proteins is determined by the rules of translation, known collectively as the genetic code. The genetic code consists of three-letter words called **'codons'** formed from a sequence of three nucleotides like ACT, CAG, TAA.

In transcription, the codons of a gene are copied into mRNA by RNA polymerase enzyme. This RNA copy is then decoded by a ribosome that reads the RNA sequence by base-pairing the mRNA to tRNA, which carries amino acids. Since there are 4 bases in 3-letter combinations, there are 64 possible codons to encode 20 amino acids. Most amino acids, therefore, have more than one possible codon. There are also three 'stop' or 'nonsense' codons signifying the end of the coding region; these are the TAA, TGA and TAG codons.

## 4.3 GENE STRUCTURE AND EXPRESSION

The eukaryotic genes exist in pieces and are termed **split genes**. The DNA sequences coding for a particular protein is **exon**. They are interrupted by one or more sequences of DNA called **introns** which do not code for protein. Introns and exons vary in length. Though the introns are different, the introns seem to have same base sequences. At their 5' end they contain GT and at 3' end AG. Split genes accommodate more DNA than is necessary for functioning of a gene.

The eukaryotic gene shows the presence of **TATA** sequence, 30 or more nucleotides from the 5', upstream of the first exon. The sequence **AATAA** is present several hundred nucleotides from the 3' end downstream.

## Transcription

The process of formation of **mRNA** transcript from DNA by **RNA polymerase** is called transcription. The **TATA box** is essential for transcription. It is known as Hogness box and represents a **promoter site** for RNA polymerase II to initiate transcription. Synthesis of mRNA proceeds in 5' to 3' direction. The actual site of initiation of transcription is located about 30 bases to the 3' side downstream of the TATA box. The transcription begins to the 5' end of the first exon which is not involved in coding for protein. After the initiation of transcription the terminal 5' nucleotide of the RNA transcript is modified by the addition of a methyl group and a triphosphate linked 7-methylguanosine residue ($m^7$Gppp). This modified base at 5' end of each RNA transcript is known as the **RNA cap** and the process is **capping**. The entire length of the gene including introns and exons are transcribed. Termination occurs at 3' end. Following termination of transcription, a tail of polyadenylic acid (AAAA) about 100 bases in length is added ( **polyadenylation**) to the 3' end of each mRNA transcript.

## mRNA Splicing

The primary transcript is converted into a functional mRNA by **splicing**. Here the intron sequences

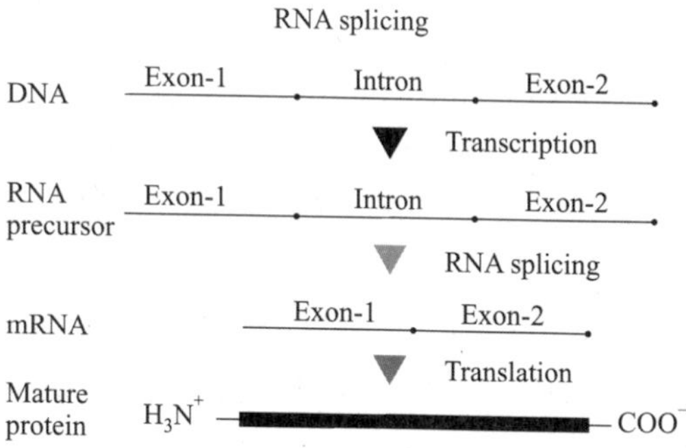


**Fig. 4.3** Split gene and splicing
(Source: www.genome.wellcome.ac.uk)

are removed and the exon sequences or joined or spliced together.

## Translation

The mature mRNA after splicing moves from nucleus to the cytoplasm to get translated into a protein. In the cytoplasm is present transfer RNA or **tRNA.** The tRNA possesses a site with specific sequence of three bases the **anticodon** which base pair with the complementary sequence of three bases in mRNA (mRNA codon). A site on tRNA is recognized by aminoacyl synthetase enzyme specific for each amino acid and these enzymes specifically attache one of twenty amino acid to the tRNA. Thus each tRNA molecule serves as an **adaptor**.It links a specific amino acid to a specific codon in the mRNA. The relationship between the DNA codons and amino acids is determined by the genetic code. The protein synthesis is initiated by a special tRNA which recognizes the AUG mRNA codon and called start codon or initiation codon. The three codons not recognized by tRNA are called stop codons or termination codons (UAA,UAG,UGA).

Polypeptide synthesis occurs in the cytoplasm on ribosomes. Each ribosome has two subunits namely 40S the smaller subunit and 60S the larger subunit. Translation begins with the formation of an **initiation complex** formed by the binding of aminoacylated initiator Met-tRNA, GTP and mRNA to 40S ribosomal subunit. **Initiation factors** elf-2 and elf-3 facilitate the process. Soon after the binding of mRNA, a 60S subunit is joined to the 40S initiation complex with the help of several other proteins and elongation of the polypeptide chain proceeds. The **elongation factors** Ef-1 and Ef-2 and enzyme peptidyl transferase play an important role in elongation process. Finally chain termination occurs when the polypeptide chain is released. This happens when the stop codons are recognized. Termination is facilitated by the **releasing factor** RF which binds to the complex and activates peptidyl transferase, releasing the peptide chain from tRNA.

## Protein Structure

The amino acid sequence of a polypeptide defines the primary structure of proteins. The secondary structure is the three dimensional form of parts of the polypeptide: the alpha helix or the beta pleated structure. Tertiary structure is the folded form of the whole polypeptide composed of different secondary structures. Quaternary structure is the final native conformation of a mutimeric protein, e.g. hemoglobin is composed of two alpha globin monomers, two beta globin monomers, one molecule of haem and an atom of ferrous iron. Collagen fibres are cables of many triple helices, each formed as a rope of three pro-alpha helices.

Structure of protein is frequently maintained by disulphide bridges between cystein residues on adjacent strands and the enzymic properties depend on the distribution of charged groups.

## Post Translational Modifications

Most of the proteins undergo modification after translation before becoming functional protein. These modifications are called **post translational modifications** so that the proteins can be folded into a specific three dimensional structure. This is often achieved by glycosylation, phosphorylation and sulfation.

Post translational modification includes removal of the N-terminal methionine and cleavage. Association occurs between similar or different polypeptides. Polypeptides destined for extracellular secretion are first glycosylated in the rough endoplasmic reticulum and Golgi apparatus of the cell. Their secretion involves a signal peptide near the N terminus that binds to a signal recognition peptide free in the cytoplasm. This links them to a receptor in the membrane of the endoplasmic reticulum. As it is synthesized the polypeptide is transferred through the membrane; when its carboxyl terminus emerges, the signal peptide is cleaved off. Polypeptides are transported to the Golgi apparatus in vesicles that bud off the endoplasmic reticulum.

**Glycosylation** is usually N linked, involving addition of a common oligosaccharide to the side chain-amino group of asparagines, as in the production of antibodies and lysozymes. Protein kinases **phosphorylate** serine and tyrosine residues. **Sulphation** of tyrosine is a signal for compartmentalization.

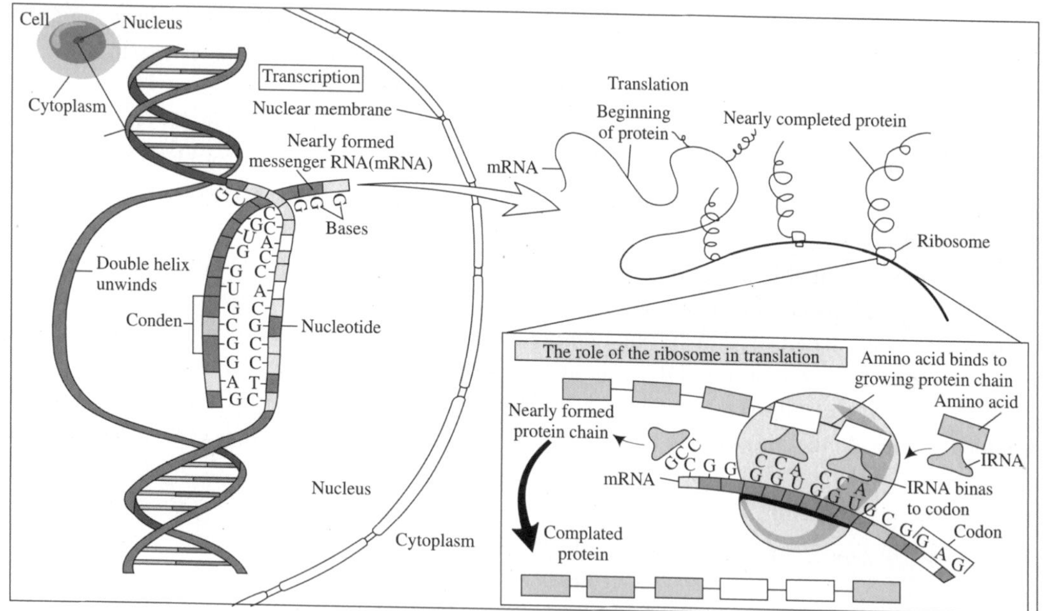


**Fig. 4.4** Protein synthesis
(Source: www.stemcells.nih.gov)

## 4.4 GENE REGULATION

The human genome is estimated to contain as many as 30,000 genes which are subjected to complex pattern of regulation. In cells all the genes are not active all the time. About 15% genes are expressed in the cells and the rest remain inactive. The activity of a specific gene varies from cell to cell. The characteristics of a cell are determined by the proteins and enzymes present which in turn are controlled by the active genes. The pattern of gene expression changes during the life time of a cell. Understanding of gene regulation is important for learning about the genetic diseases.

### Regulation of Transcription

Eukaryotic genes are regulated by altering the rate of mRNA formation. Some proteins are regulated at high rate and some at lower rate. Regulation of gene expression is achieved by the interaction of gene promoters and DNA binding proteins called **transcription factors**. Transcription of the gene by RNA polymerase is initiated by the interaction between the short DNA regulatory sequences present in the promoter that are recognized by the binding proteins called transcription factors.

Transcription is initiated by the formation of the **transcription initiation complex** (TIC) which involves binding of RNA polymerase II and a number of proteins termed transcription factors to the TATA box whose function is to locate the RNA polymerase at the correct position and initiate transcription.

Transcriptional activator proteins stimulate transcription by interacting directly with the TIC or indirectly through protein **coactivators**. The activators have two distinct functions. First they are capable of binding DNA at a specific sequence, usually a consensus sequence in a regulatory promoter. A second function is its ability to interact with other components of the transcription apparatus and influence the rate of transcription.

Some regulatory proteins act as repressors inhibiting transcription. These repressors may bind to sequences called **silencers**. These repressors may compete with activators for DNA binding sites. When a site is occupied by an activator, transcription is stimulated, but if a repressor occupies that site, no activation occurs.

**Enhancers** are capable of affecting transcription at distant promoters. In some cases activator proteins bind to enhancer and cause the DNA between enhancer and promoter to loop out, bringing the promoter and enhancer closer to one another, so that the transcriptional activator proteins are able to interact directly with the TIC. Enhancer action is limited by **insulators**. If the insulator sequence lies between the enhancer and promoter, it blocks the action of enhancer; but if the insulator lies outside the region between the two, it has no effect.

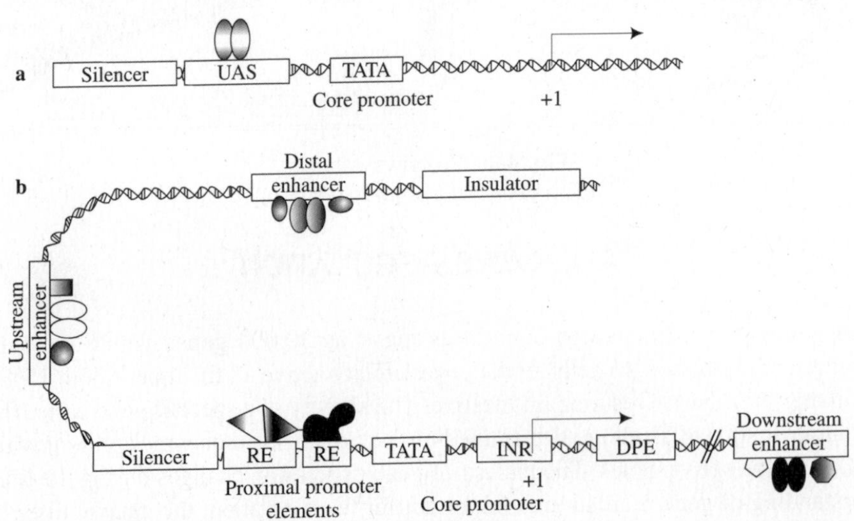


**Fig. 4.5** Transcriptional control
(Source: www.microbiology.emory.edu)

a. Simple eukaryotic transcriptional unit. A simple core promoter (TATA), upstream activator sequence (UAS) and silencer element spaced within 100–200 bp of the TATA box.
b. A complex arrangement of multiple clustered enhancer modules interspersed with silencer and insulator elements which can be located 10–50 kb either upstream or downstream of a composite core promoter containing TATA box (TATA), Initiator sequences (INR), and downstream promoter elements (DPE).

Although eukaryotes do not possess operon, several genes respond to same stimulus and this phenomenon is called coordinated gene regulation. For example many eukaryotes respond to heat and other stresses by producing **heat-shock proteins**. These are produced approximately by 20 different genes. These genes have common regulatory elements upstream of their start sites. A transcriptional activator protein binds to this regulatory element during stress and elevates transcription. Such common DNA regulatory sequences are called **response elements;** they contain short consensus sequences at varying distances from the gene being regulated.

### Gene Control Through mRNA Processing

Many eukaryotic genes undergo alternate splicing, and the regulation of splicing is probably an important means of controlling gene expression in eukaryotic cells. The T antigen gene of mammalian virus SV40 serves as a well studied example of alternate splicing. This gene is capable of encoding two different proteins, the large T and small t antigens. Which of the two proteins is produced depends on which of two alternative 5' splice sites is used during RNA splicing. The use of one 5' splice site produces mRNA that encodes the large T antigen, whereas the use of the other 5'splice site 9which is farther downstream) produces an mRNA encoding the small t antigen. **SR proteins** play a role in regulating splicing.

### Gene Control Through RNA Stability

The amount of a protein that is synthesized depends upon the amount of corresponding mRNA available for translation. This in turn depends on the rate of mRNA synthesis and mRNA degradation. Cellular RNA is degraded by ribonucleases, enzymes that specifically break down RNA. Most eukaryotic cells contain 10 or more types of ribonucleases and there are several different pathways of mRNA degradation. In one pathway, the 5'cap is first removed, followed by 5'-3' removal of nucleotides. A second pathway begins at the 3' end of the mRNA and removes nucleotides in the 3'-5' direction. In a third pathway, the mRNA can be cleaved at internal sites.

### RNA Silencing

Expression of some genes may be suppressed through RNA silencing. This is initiated by the presence of double stranded RNA that are cleaved and processed. The resulting **small interfering RNAs** (siRNA) bind to complementary sequences in mRNA and bring about their cleavage and degradation. Small interfering RNAs may also stimulate the methylation of complementary sequences in DNA.

### Translational Control

Ribosomes, aminoacyl tRNA, initiation factors and elongation factors are all required for translation of mRNA molecules. The availability of these components affects the rate of translation therefore influences gene expression. The initiation of translation may be affected by proteins that bind to specific sequences at the 5'end of mRNA and inhibit binding of ribosomes.

Many eukaryotic proteins are extensively modified after translation by the selective cleavage and trimming of amino acids from the ends by the addition of phosphates, carboxyl groups, methyl groups and carbohydrates to the protein. These modifications affect the transport, function and activity of proteins and have the capacity to affect gene expression.

CHAPTER 5

# Genetics of Human Development

## INTRODUCTION

Human life starts with the fusion of the male reproductive cell namely **sperm** and the female reproductive cell, the **ovum** resulting in **zygote**. This phenomenon of fertilization mixes up the genetic characters so that the new individual is unique. The sperm and ovum are gametes. They are unique in that they are haploid (n) cells possessing only one set of chromosomes while the other body cells are diploid (2n) since they possess two sets of chromosomes.

The gametes are produced from germ cells of the sex organs by a unique kind of cell division, the reduction division namely **meiosis**. In meiosis the chromosome number is reduced to half. The zygote divides repeatedly by mitosis to produce millions of body cells by **mitosis** which are diploid.

## 5.1 REPRODUCTIVE CELLS

### Sperm

Sperms are tiny male gametes consisting of a head, middle piece and a tail. It contains a nucleus with the chromosomes plus mitochondria for energy and a tail for movement. The human sperm is about 0.06 mm in length. There is a protrusion in the anterior end, the acrosome, contains enzymes helping in fertilization. There are 250 million sperm in one ejaculate of a fertile male.

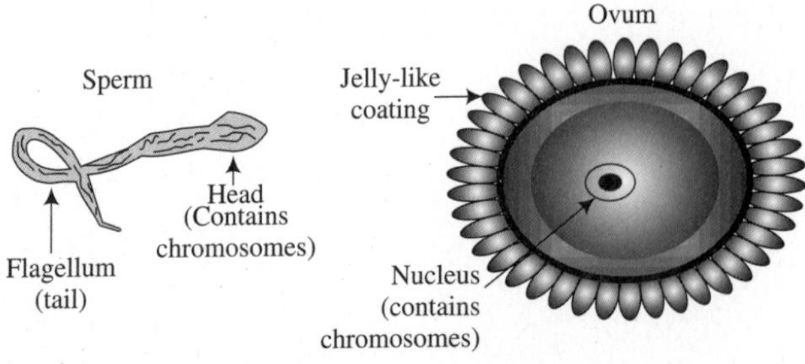


**Fig. 5.1** Structure of sperm and ovum
(Source: www.anthropalomar.edu)

Sperms are produced by **spermatogenesis**. The spermatogonium is the diploid cell of the testis that gives rise to the sperms. The spermatogonia accumulate cytoplasm and replicate DNA and are called primary spermatocytes. Each primary spermatocyte undergoes meiotic division I, forming two haploid cells called secondary spermatocyte. These divide by meiosis II producing two equal sized spermatids. The spermatids undergo specialization developing tail resulting in a tadpole shaped sperm or spermatozoa.

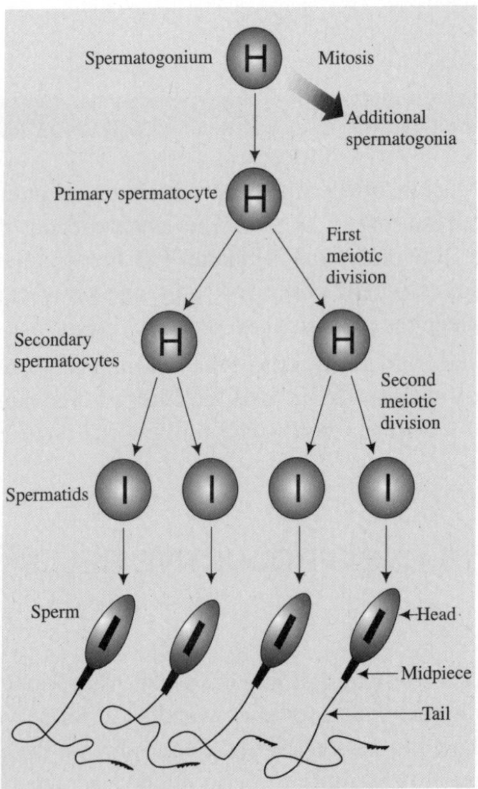


**Fig. 5.2** Spermatogenesis
(Source : www.users.rcn.com)

### Ovum

Ovum is produced by **oogenesis** from the ovary the female reproductive organ. Human ovum measures about 0.1mm. It is surrounded by the membrane zona pellucida. The ovum is produced from a diploid cell the oogonium. It grows, accumulates cytoplasm and replicates its DNA and forms primary oocyte. The primary oocyte divides unequally into a small cell with very little cytoplasm, called a polar body and a larger cell called a secondary oocyte. These cells are haploid and are surrounded by follicular cells. The polar body again divides equally to produce two polar bodies. The secondary oocyte divides unequally to form a small polar body and a large ovum. The polar bodies are often absorbed and they do not play a role in development. At birth, in a female the number of ova is predetermined and they remain in arrested condition. After puberty the cell division continues and oocytes are released regularly each month in response to hormone activity. This is termed ovulation. A female ovulates about 400 oocytes between puberty and menopause. Only few of these are used by sperms in fertilization to produce new human life.

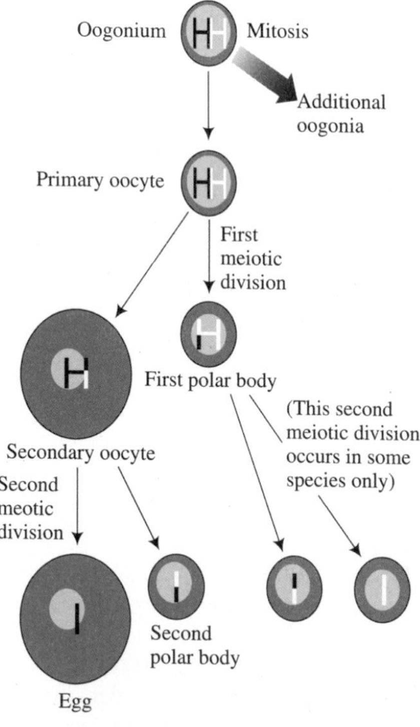


**Fig. 5.3** Oogenesis
(Source : www.users.rcn.com)

## 5.2 FERTILIZATION AND DEVELOPMENT

Millions of sperms are deposited in the female vagina during sexual intercourse. A sperm can remain alive for 3 days. An ouvm can be fertilized 12 to 24 hours after ovulation. Sperms are chemically activated by a process called **capacitation**. The ovum secretes substances that attract the sperm. The sperm migrates up the female reproductive tract with its tail. When the sperm touches the follicle cells of the secondary oocyte, the acrosome bursts releasing enzymes. When the membranes of sperm and ovum meet the **fertilization** or conception begins. Only one sperm fuses with the ovum. After 12 hours of sperm penetration the chromosomes of the sperm and ovum called **pronuclei** fuse. Fertilization is complete and the fertilized ovum is called a **zygote**.

## Implantation

After 24 hours the zygote undergoes repeated cell division called **cleavage** and the resulting cells are blastomeres. A solid ball of 16 cells is formed and the preembryo is called morula. A cavity with fluid appears in the centre and a **blastocyst** is formed. The group of cells in the blastocyst is termed **inner cell mass** (ICM) from which the embryo develops. After a week the blastocyst burries into the lining of the uterus and the event is called **implantation**. The outermost cells of the human pre-embryo are called trophoblast which secretes the **human chorionic gonadotropin** (HCG). This hormone prevents mensuration. HCG detected in a female's urine or blood indicates pregnancy.

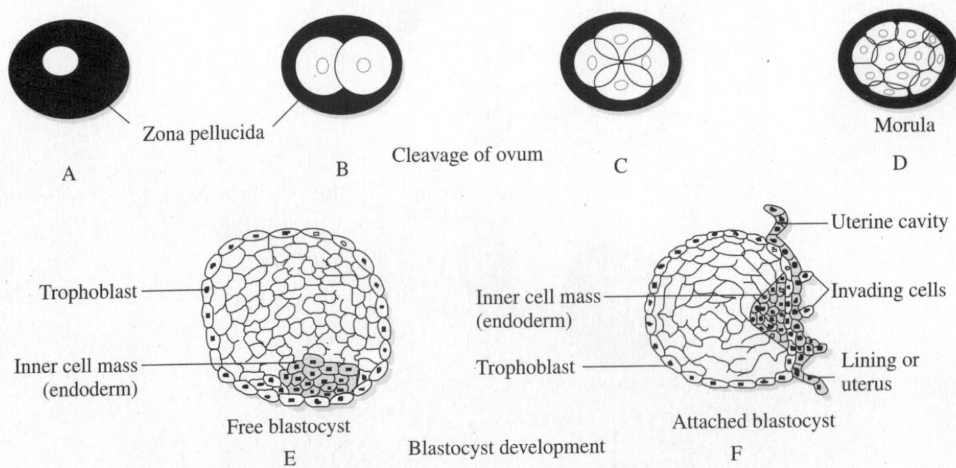


**Fig. 5.4** Early embryonic development (Source: www. biology.kenyon.edu)

In the second week of prenatal development the **amniotic cavity** appears between the inner cell mass and the outer cells. The inner cell mass forms two layers, the outer one lying near the amniotic cavity is the ectoderm and the inner layer closer to the blastocyst cavity is the endoderm. Later a middle layer, the mesoderm appears. This three layered structure is gastrula and the cell layers are called primary germ layers. It is now considered as an **embryo**. Cells in the specific germ layers later become part of particular organ systems due to differential expression of genes.

When the embryo is 3 to 8 weeks of pregnancy organs develop. By the third week after conception, finger like projections called **chorionic villi** extend from cells of the embryo lying near the uterine wall. The blood system of the mother and embryo are separate but nutrients and oxygen diffuse across the chorionic villi from the maternal circulation to the embryo and wastes leave the embryo and enter mother's circulation to be excreted out. By 10 weeks a placenta is fully formed connecting the mother and the fetus. Hormones are secreted by the placenta and maintain pregnancy. There is a yolk sac manufacturing blood cells and an allantois which gives rise to umbilical blood vessels. The umbilical cord is formed around these blood vessels and attaches to the center of the placenta. At the end of the embryonic period, the yolk sac shrinks and the amniotic sac swells with fluid that cushions the embryo.

In the third week, a primitive streak appears along the back of the embryo, forming an axis around which the organs are organized. The primitive streak gives rise to a notochord which forms the basic structure for the skeleton. A reddish bulge containing the heart appears and it starts beating by day 18. By fourth week blood vessels, lungs and kidneys appear. The embryo now develops a distinct head, jaws, eyes, ears and nose. The digestive system appears as a hollow long tube and the embryo is ¼ inch long. There is the appearance of a neural tube that will house the central nervous system. Arms and legs begin to form as buds. By the fifth week the embryo's head becomes very large. The eyes open. By the seventh and eighth week a skeleton appears. At eighth week of gestation, the embryo has all the structures that will present at birth. It is now a fetus. Soon, as the nerves and muscles coordinate, the fetus will move its arms and legs.

Sex is determined at conception, when an X or Y bearing sperm fertilizes the ovum. The SRY gene in the Y chromosome determines the maleness. At the sixth week the male hormone stimulates the development of male reproductive organs from an undifferentiated structure. In the absence of male hormone the undifferentiated structures develop into female reproductive organs. By week 12, the fetus sucks it's thumb, kicks and baby teeth appears. It breathes amniotic fluid in and out, and excretes and urinates. Now the first trimester is over. By the fourth month, the fetus develops hair, eyebrows, eye lashes and nails. The vocal cords are formed by 18 weeks. The fetus takes up the characteristic curled position by the end of the fifth month. By the end of second trimester the fetus turns pink with wrinkled skin. The fetus is now 9 inches long. The brain develops completely at the final trimester. All the organ systems mature.

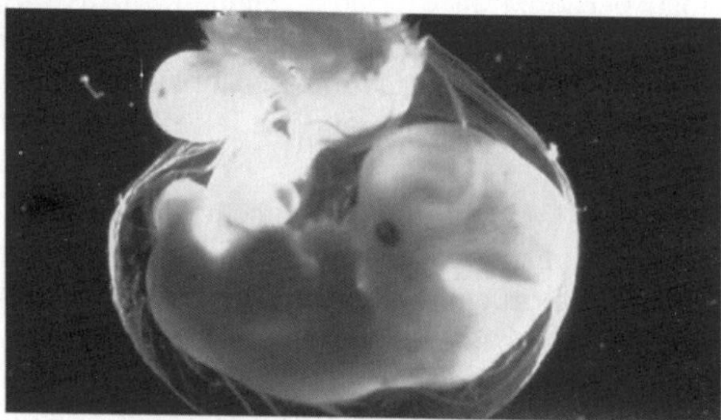

**Fig. 5.5** Human embryo
(Source: www.scienceclassified.com)

Approximately after 266 days after fertilization the baby is ready to be born. From the 9$^{th}$ week to 38 weeks the fetus will increase in weight and in length. A 26 week-old fetus may survive if born prematurely. With improved technology it is possible to keep alive some babies born even with a weight of 500 g and 22 weeks old.

## 5.3 SENSITIVE PERIODS IN DEVELOPMENT AND CONGENITAL DEFECTS

The most crucial and sensitive developmental period extends between weeks three and eight. At this time major organ system begins to take form and the presence of alcohol, drugs, viruses or radiation may lead to malformation. These agents are called **teratogens** (teratos = monster; gen = producing). Any agent interfering with the development of an organism can cause malformations in the embryo. The study of how environmental agents disrupt normal development is called teratology.

Congenital (at birth) abnormalities and demise of embryos and fetuses prior to birth are caused by various factors. Those abnormalities caused by genetic events such as mutations and chromosomal aberrations are called malformations. Abnormalities due to exogenous agents such as chemicals, radiation, hypothermia and viruses are called disruption.

Most congenital defects are due to a complex interaction of genetic information and environmental factors. Examples are cleft lip, cleft palate and spina bifida (cleft spine).

Spina bifida affects 1 of every 1,000 newborn, occurs when one or more spinal vertebrae fail to close and the spinal cord with nerves bulge through the cleft. Most spina bifida babies also suffer from mental retardation caused by hydrocephalus, an abnormal accumulation of fluids in the brain.

Although genes play a role in some congenital defects, many birth defects are caused by environment agents called teratogens. For example, if a woman is infected with rubella virus (German measles) while she is pregnant, the embryo may develop heart defects or suffer damage to its eyes or ears. **Cytomegalovirus** infection is always fatal but infection of later embryos can lead to blindness, cerebral palsy and mental retardation. *Toxoplama gondii* causes brain and eye defects in the fetus.

A tragic example of a drug induced congenital defect is caused by **thalidomide**, a tranquilizer that was used by pregnant mother in 1950 to 1960 to reduce anxiety in expectant mothers. Thalidomide a mild sedative caused an enormous anomalies called **phocomelia** (limbless). Thalidomide is a potent teratogen in human beings, and thousands of women who took this drug early in pregnancy gave birth to children who had abnormal or missing limbs (armless and legless). The drug was found to be teratogenic only during days 34 to 50 after last mensuration and this period is the period of susceptibility.

Methotrexate, a drug used in cancer treatment, trimethodiane, an anticonvulsant, phenytoin and anticoagulants such as warfarin are also teratogenic. Quinine, the anti malarial drug can cause deafness in the fetus. Nicotine and caffeine in women who smoke 20 cigarettes/day are likely to have infants that are smaller than those born to women who do not smoke.

Pesticides and organic mercury compounds have caused neurological and behavioral abnormalities in infants whose mothers have ingested them during pregnancy. A tragic incident occurred in 1965, when a Japanese firm dumped mercury into a lake, where it was ingested by the fishes, which were eaten by pregnant women in the village of Minamata. The congenital brain damage and blindness in the children resulted in Minamata disease.

Retinoic acids are analogues of Vitamin A. 13-cis-retinoic acid is a treatment for severe cystic acne. The pregnant woman when exposed to retinoic acid, gave birth to malformed infants which had characteristic pattern of abnormalities, including absent or defective ears, absent or small jaws, cleft palate and abnormalities of central nervous system.

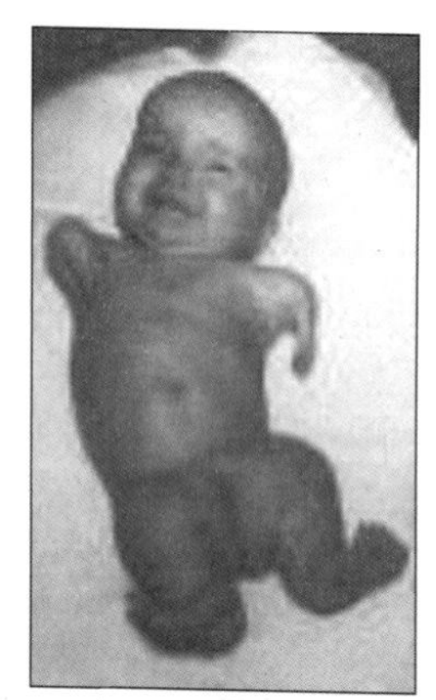

**Fig. 5.6** Thalidomide tragedy (Source: www.medicineworld.org)

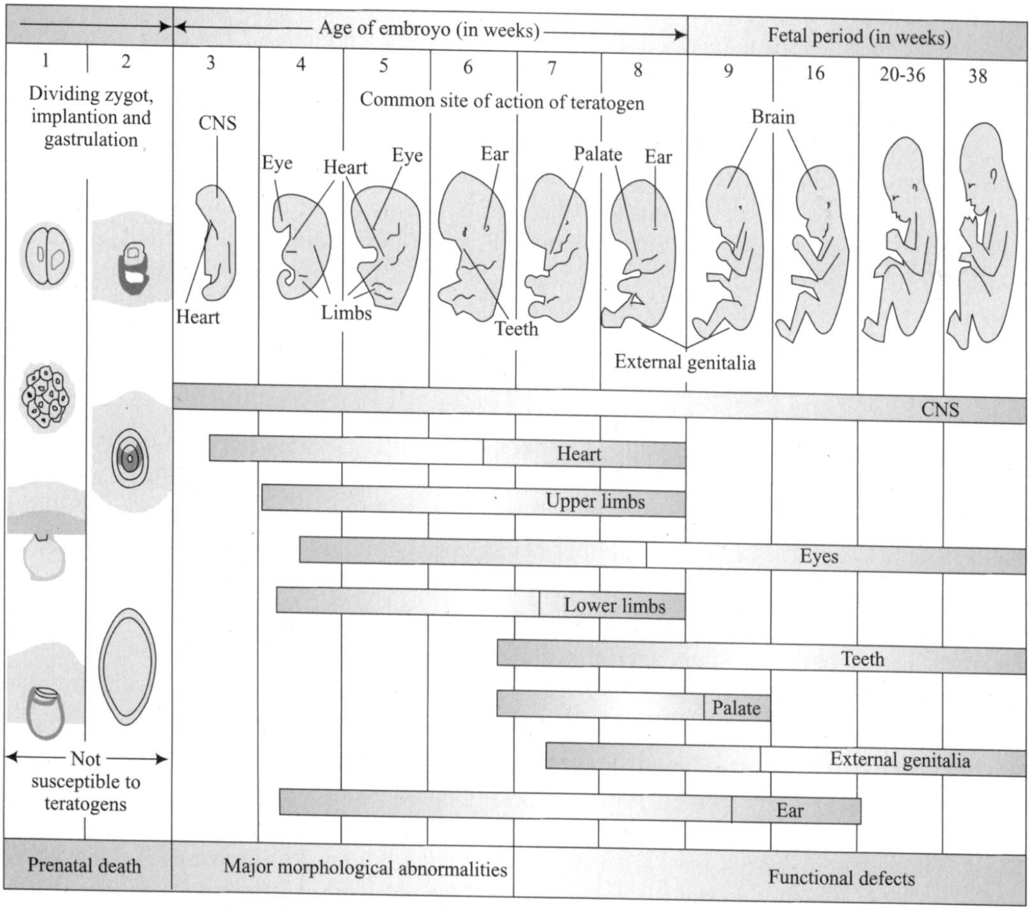

Alcohol is another teratogen; it can cause serious physical defects and produce fetal alcohol syndrome (FAS). This is characterized by small head size, indistinct ridge between nose and mouth, a narrow upper lip and a low nose bridge. The brain is also smaller. Severe mental retardation occurs. Their mean IQ is 68. Because of the uncertanity about which substances are teratogenic, pregnant women are advised to forego taking drugs of any kind, including alcohol, caffeine, aspirin and tobacco.

Age of embroyo (in weeks)
Fetal period (in weeks)
1 2 3 4 5 6 7 8 9 16 20-36 38
Dividing zygot, implantion and gastrulation
Common site of action of teratogen
CNS
Heart
Eye
Heart
Eye
Limbs
Ear
Teeth
Palate
Ear
External genitalia
Brain
CNS
Heart
Upper limbs
Eyes
Lower limbs
Teeth
Palate
External genitalia
Ear
Not susceptible to teratogens
Prenatal death
Major morphological abnormalities
Functional defects

**Fig. 5.7** Human embryonic development and critical periods (Source: www.embryology.med.unsw.edu.au)

## 5.4 CHROMOSOMAL ABNORMALITIES AND SPONTANEOUS ABORTIONS

Abortion is defined as termination of pregnancy before 20 to 22 weeks of development or when embryonic weight is less than 400-500 gms. Abortion can be spontaneous or induced. As many as 15% of all confirmed pregnancies spontaneously terminate in utero. A woman is termed a habitual aborter when she records three or more miscarriages. 90% of spontaneous abortions occur in first trimester of pregnancy and the embryo is usually less than 8 weeks old. When cells from spontaneously aborted embryos are examined, at least half of them have observable chromosomal abnormalities of various kinds. In the youngest abortuses (4 weeks old) the frequency of abnormalities is 90% and among those aged 5-8 weeks it is about 60% and those of 9-12 weeks of age, it ranges from 12-32%. The single most common chromosomal aberration is 45X. Polyploids are the next more frequent class of abnormalities, while structural abnormalities occur in only 2% of spontaneous fetal deaths. The rest of them also may have genetic defects, such as small translocation or inversions which cannot be detected under microscope. The high frequency of chromosomal abnormalities indicates how often mistakes occur in meiosis. The high frequency of spontaneous abortions also shows that nature has evolved mechanisms to recognize and eliminate genetically abnormal embryos. Most embryos with an extra chromosome do not survive to term; and an exception is 21trisomy, which results in Down syndrome. Roughly 1% of all recognized pregnancies end in stillbirths. Anything that is born dead or nearly dying at birth is called still births, whose observed rate of chromosomal abnormalities is about one-tenth of that found in spontaneous abortuses. Among stillbirths trisomy18 is the most common aberration. A striking maternal age effect has been noted in these studies. About 35% of still births and neonatal deaths from mothers over age 40 had chromosomal aberrations, whereas only 6% of those born to mother under 40 showed chromosomal abnormalities.

Miscarriage (loss of baby) occurs in the first 6 months of pregnancy. 75% of miscarriages occur during the first trimester. 3% of miscarriages take place during second trimester. Miscarriage is caused by the fertilized egg when it fails to undergo chromosomal divisions properly. More than 50% of miscarriages are caused by chromosomal abnormality. Maternal age also causes an increase in the risk of miscarriage. Miscarriages are sometimes due to the result of the fetus inability to maintain its attachment to the placenta, either because of hormonal imbalance or a weak uterus unable to support the weight of the growing fetus. The first sign of miscarriage is vaginal bleeding.

Neonatal death is the death of new born baby. 35% of still births and neonatal death from mother over age 40 had karyotypic aberrations and only 6% of those born to mothers under 40 showed chromosomal abnormalities. Among the various abnormal karyotypes, the common ones are autosomal trisomies, Klinefelter syndrome and Turner syndrome.

If either the egg or the sperm has an abnormal number of chromosomes, the embryo may abort spontaneously early in development. When embryonic cells undergo hundreds of cell divisions, and each time the cells chromosomes must undergo mitosis and the cells must divide with precision. Thus, genetic errors may arise in chromosomes during development of the embryo, causing it to abort. Finally, during the many month of embryonic development, genes must be switched off and on and expressed in a precise sequence if abnormal development is not to result.

Medical illness like congenital cardiac disease, jaundice and renal disease in a pregnant woman may also cause fetal loss. In pregnant woman the incidence of fetal loss may be extremely high with coexistent hypertension and uncontrolled diabetes mellitus. Women who have repeated abortion lack a key serum-blocking antibody that is supposed to protect the fetus from rejection by the mother. The blocking factor belongs to the IgG class and acts to protect the fetus from maternal antibodies. Reduction in the production of progesterone, the luteal hormone may result in fetal loss. The hormonal imbalance may occur due to oophoritis (inflammation of ovary), bacterial or Trichomonas infection of the uterus. Many of the psychogenic causing factors could bring about habitual abortion.

The occurrence of trisomy in live births and spontaneous abortions increases with the age of the mother (maternal age effect). Researches indicate that a mother of 35 years has more risk carrying a child affected by Down syndrome. The risk is 3% higher compare to mother of 25 years. Seven other chromosomal disorders are also of higher frequencies when the pregnant woman is above 35 years.

## 5.5 TWINS

Humans normally bear only one offspring at a time. But some times multiple birth occurs. Twins result from the simultaneous intrauterine development of two embryos. Twins are of three kinds.

### *1. Identical or Monozygotic Twins (MZ)*

They are derived from a single fertilized ovum and accquires identical chromosomal constitution. They develop from a single blastocyst, contained within a common chorionic sac and share a common placenta. The umbilical cord and the amniotic cavity also may not be separate. The twins have similar features, same sex and identical blood group.

### *2. Non Identical or Fraternal or Dizygotic Twins (DZ)*

They are due to the simultaneous fertilization of two ova from the same or different ovaries by separate sperms. Each has its own chromosomal constitution, chorionic sac and placenta. The sex and blood group may or may not be the same. They resemble one another but not identical

### *3. Conjoined Twins*

These are true twins who are joined with each other. Such double monsters are termed as Siamese twins. They arise from the incomplete separation of the two embryos developed from a single zygote.

### Twin Studies in Genetic Analysis

MZ have all their genes in common. Their genotypes are identical. DZ have 50% of their genes common like any other sisters and brothers. MZ twins provide good opportunity to evaluate the roles of genes and environment in the development of a trait. A unique opportunity is provided by those rare identical twins who have been raised apart since infancy. In this situation the environmental effects would be more varied on twins reared apart than on those raised together, the contribution of environmental factors to the expression of a trait can be shown. A pair of identical twins thus gives the opportunity to study the expression of the same genotype in a similar environment (monozygotic twins reared together) and the expression of same genotype in different environments (MZ reared apart).

Two identical twins should always show the same trait if that trait is entirely based on hereditary factors. For example MZ will have identical blood groups. If the two members of a twin pair are alike with regard to a certain trait then they are said to be **concordant**. Among MZ, 100% would be concordant with regard to ABO blood type. Members of a twin pair are **discordant** if they differ with respect to a given trait. If 1 pair of MZ under study is discordant, the operation of environmental factors is indicated. If MZ and DZ are showing similar concordance value then the strong role of environment is indicated. If only heredity is involved then MZ should show a high concordance. Suppose in a study of a trait, MZ show 80% concordance and DZ show 20% concordance for the same trait, it indicates a strong hereditary component for the trait. If both MZ and DZ approximately show the same amount of concordance such as 70%, then the greater importance of the environment would be indicated.

In a study on eye color a concordance value of 99.6% was obtained for MZ revealing a strong hereditary component for this trait. The susceptibility to measles when studied showed 95% concordance for MZ and 87% concordance for DZ indicating the environmental influence on this condition. The concordance values for stomach cancer suggest a hereditary component since a significant difference between the MZ and DZ was noted (27% for MZ and 4% for DZ) but a large environmental component (73% of MZ are discordant).

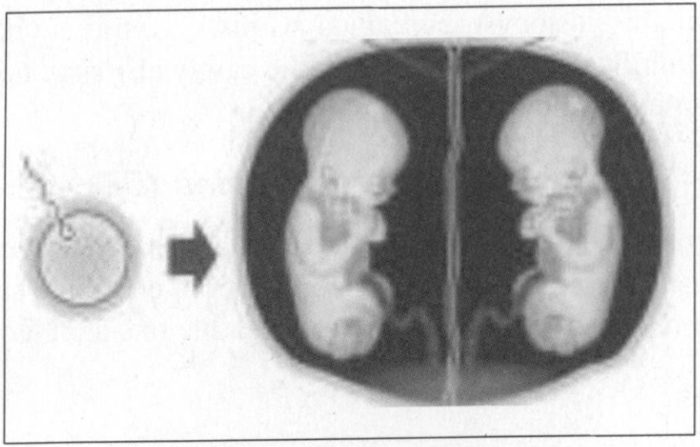

**Fig. 5.8** Monozygotic twins
(Source: www.mombaby.com)

## 5.6 AGING PROCESS

Aging is an uninterrupted continuation phase in normal development. It is in a sense, programmed death in which birth is followed by maturation, postmaturation and finally death. Aging process is the result of a combination of mechanisms that interact to cause cell dysfunction, cell death, tissue dysfunction and death. Generally, following birth, there is a period of growth and development leading to reproductive maturity. During this process, which is programmed in the genetic material, changes in the synthesis of gene products occur. Patterns of hormones, enzymes and antibodies change as a person enters postmaturation period. There are alterations in the protein synthesis pattern resulting in the alterations of cell environment. These altered environments lead to deteriorating functions and the final phase is senescence (old age) and death.

The life spans are more are less fixed for each species is strong evidence that aging is genetically controlled. The individual variation throws light on the environmental influence on aging. Each cell type has definite number of cell divisions in its life time. Once that number has been reached, the cells deteriorate and die. This is referred as **Hayflick limit** and is attributed to the cells in culture. For example, a human embryonic connective tissue cell divides 50 times and a connective tissue cell culture after birth divides about 30 times.

Biologists believe that aging is controlled by a developmental 'clock'. One such developmental model is called the codon-restriction model of aging. According to this model, at different developmental stages, the proportions of different tRNA molecules and the synthetase enzymes that link them to amino acids undergo series of changes. This change alters the sequential gene expression controlled by translation, altering the codon-producing capacities of the genes. There is sequential activation and repression of selected gene activity. The appearance and disappearance of the gene products control the aging process.

Mutations and repair mechanisms may play a role in the aging process. Somatic mutations may accumulate giving rise to clones of abnormal cells that has negative impact. The DNA repairing capacity of the cell also reduces resulting in the occurrence of cancers.

Another model proposed to explain aging is termed error-catastrophe model of aging. This model suggests that errors occur in the synthesis of polypeptides and these altered polypeptides trigger other errors, resulting in cascading effect. The accumulation of errors leads to cell dysfunction and ultimately death.

There are some genetically caused premature aging syndromes. The most popular one is Progeria syndrome. It is a dominant disorder. The person with this disease has an average life span of about 11 years but looks like an old person. There is no single gene responsible for aging syndrome instead it is controlled by a complex series of genes interacting with one another.

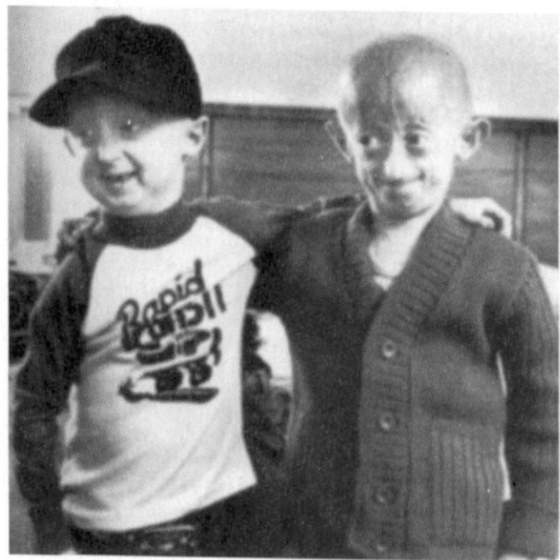

**Fig. 5.9** Progeria syndrome
(Source: www.unc.edu)

CHAPTER 6

# Human Pedigrees and Inheritance Patterns

## INTRODUCTION

The study of inherited Mendelian traits in humans must rely on observations made while working with individual families. Classical cross fertilization breeding experiments as performed by Mendel are not allowed in humans. Human geneticists are not allowed to selectively breed for the traits they wish to study. One of most powerful tools in human genetic studies is **pedigree analysis**. When human geneticists first began to publish family studies, they used a variety of symbols and conventions. Now there are agreed upon standards for the construction of pedigrees.

Pedigree analysis is one of the best methods of analyzing inheritance. It determines the mode of inheritance of a trait. Pedigree is a chart or diagram representing the ancestral history of an individual. It is a shorthand or graphic representation of the details of a family. Individuals are characterized according to their sex, their generation, and their biologic relationship to each other.

Typically, a three-generation pedigree is obtained, beginning with the patient. For example, if an infant is being evaluated, the pedigree should include sibs, parents, aunts and uncles, nieces and nephews and grandparents. When evaluating an adult, it is often helpful to expand the pedigree to include children and grandchildren. If a pattern of illness emerges, it is important to extend the family history back as many generations as possible to include any additional affected relatives.

## 6.1 FACTUAL AND HEALTH INFORMATION TO INCLUDE IN A PEDIGREE

- Age/birth date
- Age of death
- Cause of death
- Pregnancy complications (e.g., miscarriage, stillbirth, pregnancy termination)
- Infertility vs. number of children by choice
- Relevant health information (i.e., height, weight, etc.)
- Affected/unaffected status (defined by shading of symbols in key/legend)
- Ethnic background
- Consanguinity
- Date when pedigree was drawn
- Name of person who provided the data

## 6.2 SYMBOLS APPLIED

Males are always represented by square symbols, females with circular symbols. A line drawn between a square and a circle represents a mating of that male and female. Two lines drawn between

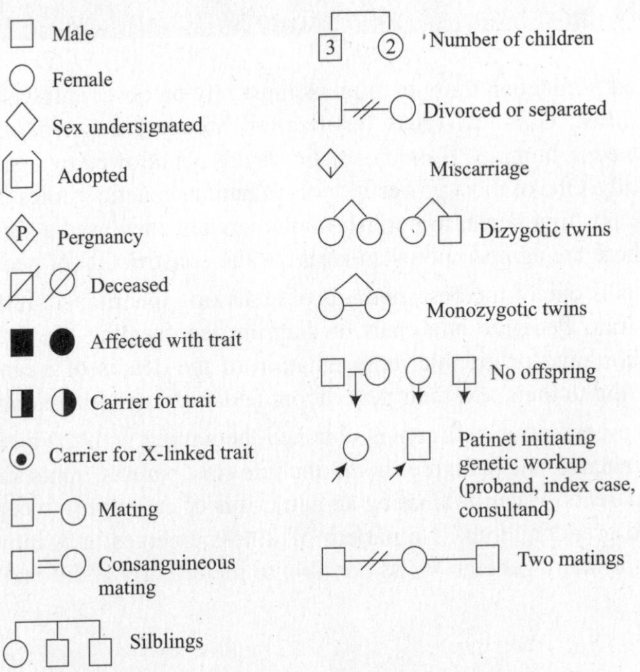


**Fig. 6.1** Symbols applied in a pedigree (Source: www.uic.edu)

a square and a circle indicate a consanguineous mating, the two individuals are related, usually second cousins or closer relatives. When possible, the square should be placed on the left and the circle on the right of the mating line. Generations are connected by a vertical line extending down from the mating line to the next generation. Children of a mating are connected to a horizontal line, called the sib-ship line, by short vertical lines. The children of a sib-ship are always listed in order of birth, the oldest being on the left. Normal individuals are represented by an open square or circle, depending upon the gender, and affected individuals by a solid square or circle. Each generation is numbered to the left of the sib-ship line with Roman Numerals. Individuals in each generation are numbered sequentially, beginning on the left, with Arabic Numerals. For example the third individual in the second generation would be identified as individual II-3.

## 6.3 INHERITANCE PATTERNS

### a. Autosomal Dominant Inheritance

The pattern of autosomal dominant inheritance is perhaps the easiest type of Mendelian inheritance to recognize in a pedigree. One allele responsible for a trait is all that is required for the expression of the phenotype.

The features for this pattern are given below:

With the understanding that almost all affected individuals are heterozygotes, and that in most matings involving a person with an autosomal dominant trait the other partner will be homozygous normal, there are four hallmarks of autosomal dominant inheritance.

1. Generally every affected individual has an affected biological parent.
2. The transmission of the trait is from generation to generation without skipping of generations.
3. Males and females have an equally likely chance of inheriting the mutant allele and being affected.

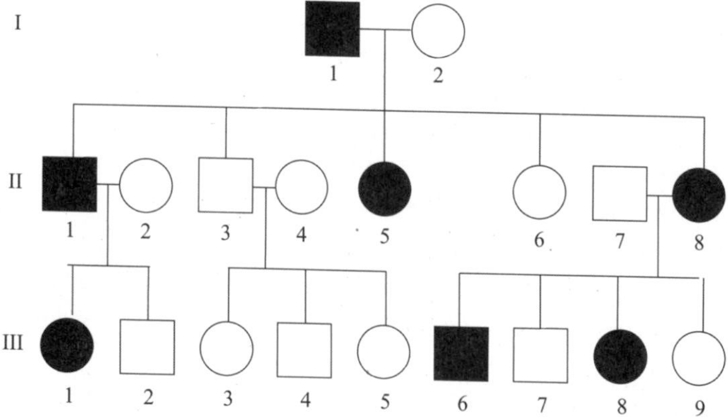


**Fig. 6.2** Sample pedigree for autosomal dominant inheritance

4. In the mating between an affected heterozygote to a normal, each child has 50% chance to inherit the abnormal allele and be affected and a 50% chance to inherit the normal allele.

The family represented in the above pedigree is a good example of how autosomal dominant diseases appear in a pedigree. Each of the four hallmarks of autosomal dominant inheritance is fulfilled. About 50% of the offsprings of an affected individual are affected (the recurrence risk is 50%). Normal offspring II-3 of affected individuals have all normal offsprings.

**Examples**

1. **Achondroplasia** (dwarfism): AA = homozygous dominant is lethal (fatal spontaneous abortion of fetus). Aa = dwarfism. aa = no dwarfism. 99.96% of all people in the world are homozygous recessive (aa).
2. **Polydactyly** (extra fingers or toes): PP or Pp = extra digits, aa = 5 digits. 98% of all people in the world are homozygous recessive (pp).

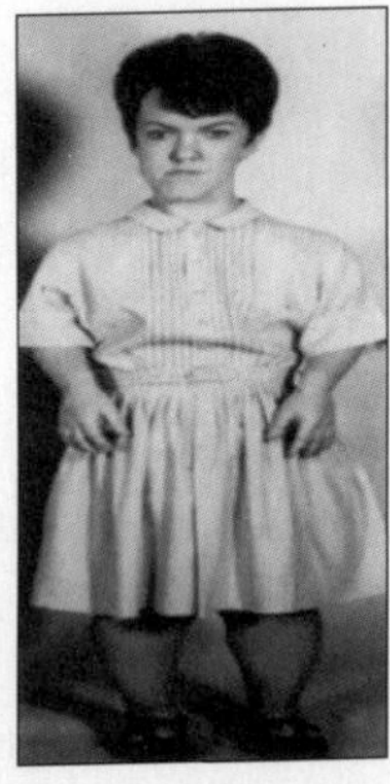

**Fig. 6.3** Achondroplasia
(Source: www.nature.com)

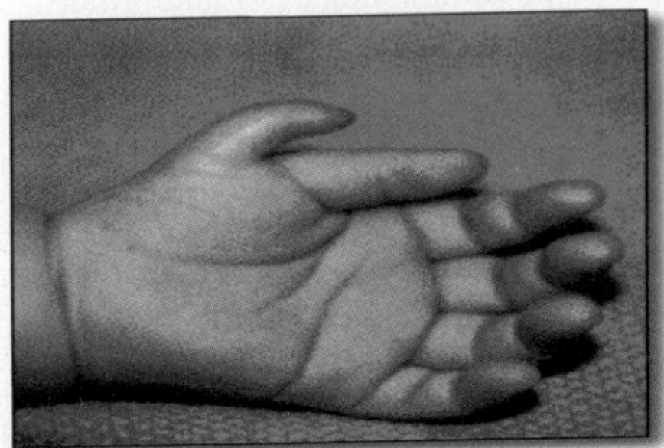

**Fig. 6.4** Polydactyly
(Source: www.nature.com)

3. **Progeria** (very premature aging): Spontaneous mutation of one gene creates a dominant mutation that rapidly accelerates aging.

### *b. Autosomal Recessive Inheritance*

The first, and most important, thing to remember about autosomal recessive inheritance is that most, if not all, affected individuals have parents with normal phenotypes.

There are four hallmarks of autosomal recessive inheritance:

1. Males and females are equally likely to be affected.
2. On average, the recurrence risk to the unborn sibling of an affected individual is 1/4.
3. The trait is characteristically found in siblings, not parents of affected or the offspring of affected.
4. Parents of affected children may be related and a consanguineous mating is involved.

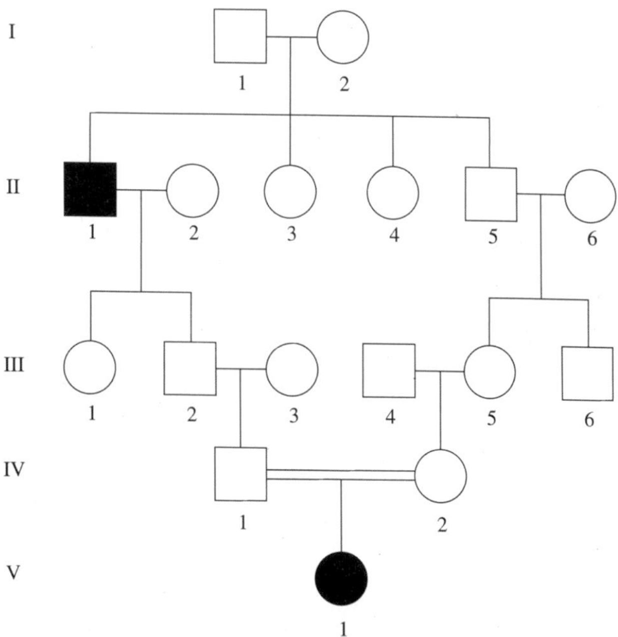


**Fig. 6.5** Pedigree for autosomal recessive inheritance

The above pedigree illustrates four hallmarks of autosomal recessive inheritance. I-1 and I-2 are unrelated, yet they produced an affected offspring (affected offspring have normal parents). By chance, they both must have been carriers.

When consanguinity is involved, i.e., matings between related individuals, in the production of an affected child the assignment of probabilities changes, especially in the rarer autosomal recessive diseases. Consanguinity introduces the possibility of one founding parent being a carrier, with the recessive allele being passed through carrier offspring and produces an affected homozygous offspring some generations later. When an affected child is produced as the result of a consanguineous mating, those individuals in the direct line of descent are most probably carriers and those from outside the family are most probably normal homozygotes. V-1 is affected with an autosomal recessive disease. Her parents are second cousins. IV-1 and IV-2 must both be carriers since they produced an affected child. (The child must have received a recessive allele from each of her parents.) III-2 is an obligate carrier. Her father was affected, and hence, a homozygote for the recessive allele. III-5 must also be heterozygotes since IV-2 had to get her recessive allele from one of her parent, and the chance of III-6 being a carrier is less than 1 in 50. I-1 and I-2 must have been carriers since they produced an affected offspring, II-1.

**Examples**

1. **Cystic fibrosis:** Homozygous recessives (*cc*) have cystic fibrosis – body cannot make needed chloride channel, high concentrations of extracellular chloride causes mucous to build up, infections and pneumonia. Diet, antibiotics and treatment can extend life to 25 years or more. Cystic fibrosis: Cc carriers are resistant to cholera (4% of caucasians is a carrier *Aa*).

2. **Tay–Sachs disease:** Enzyme that breaks down brain lipids is non-functional in homozygous recessives (*tt*). Buildup of lipids causes death by age 2-3. Tay-Sachs: Tt carriers are thought to be more resistant to tuberculosis.
3. **Sickle cell disease:** The most common inherited disease of African-Americans (1:400 affected). Homozygous recessives (*ss*) make abnormal form of hemoglobin that deforms red blood cells and causes a cascade of symptoms (clogging of blood vessels, organ damage and kidney failure). Sickle cell disease: Ss carriers are resistant to malaria (10% African-Americans are carriers *Ss*).

### *c. Sex Linked Inheritance*

If the gene for a particular trait or disease lies on the X chromosome, the disease is said to be X-linked. The inheritance pattern for X-linked inheritance differs from autosomal inheritance only because the X chromosome has no homologous chromosome in the male, the male has an X and a Y chromosome. Very few genes have been discovered on the Y chromosome.

The inheritance pattern follows the pattern of segregation of the X and Y chromosomes in meiosis and fertilization. A male child always gets his X from one of his mother's two X's and his Y chromosome from his father. X-linked genes are never passed from father to son. A female child always gets the father's X chromosome and one of the two X's of the mother. An affected female must have an affected father. Males are always hemizygous for X linked traits, that is, they can never be heterozygotes or homozygotes. They are never carriers. A single dose of a mutant allele will produce a mutant phenotype in the male, whether the mutation is dominant or recessive. On the other hand, females must be either homozygous for the normal allele, heterozygous, or homozygous for the mutant allele, just as they are for autosomal loci.

### *c.i. X Linked dominant inheritance*

When an X-linked gene is said to express dominant inheritance, it means that a single dose of the mutant allele will affect the phenotype of the female.

A recessive X-linked gene requires two doses of the mutant allele to affect the female phenotype. The following are the hallmarks of X-linked dominant inheritance:

1. The trait is never passed from father to son.
2. All daughters of an affected male and a normal female are affected. All sons of an affected male and a normal female are normal.
3. Matings of affected females and normal males produce 1/2 the sons affected and 1/2 the daughters affected.
4. In the general population, females are more likely to be affected than males, even if the disease is not lethal in males.

The following Punnett Squares explain the first three hallmarks of X-linked dominant inheritance. X represents the X chromosome with the normal allele, XA represents the X chromosome with the mutant dominant allele, and Y represents the Y chromosome. Note that the affected father never passes the trait to his sons but passes it to all of his daughters, since the heterozygote is affected for dominant traits. On the other hand, an affected female passes the disease to half of her daughters and half of her sons.

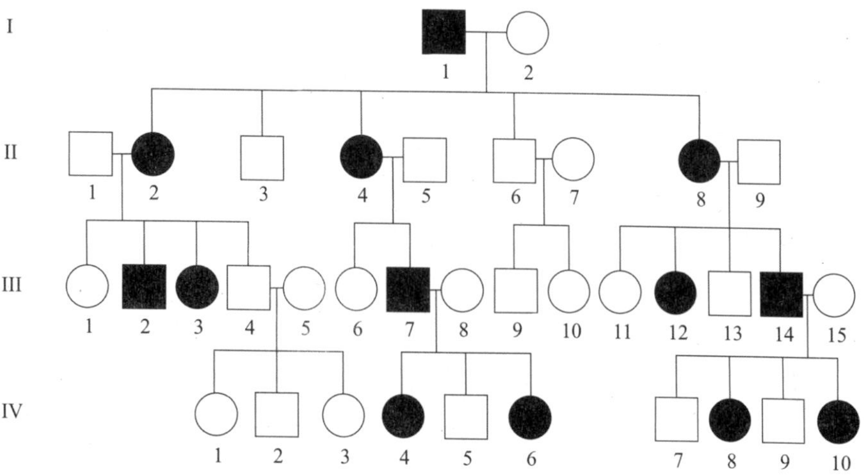


**Fig. 6.6** Pedigree for X-linked dominant inheritance

**Table 6.1.a** Mating between affected father & normal mother

| | | *Father's Gametes* | |
|---|---|---|---|
| | | $X^A$ | Y |
| Mother's | X | $XX^A$ | XY |
| Gametes | X | $XX^A$ | XY |

**Table 6.1.b** Mating between affected mother & normal father

| | | *Father's Gametes* | |
|---|---|---|---|
| | | X | Y |
| Mother's | $X^A$ | $X^AX$ | $X^AY$ |
| Gametes | X | XX | XY |

Males are usually more severely affected than females because in each affected female there is one normal allele producing a normal gene product and one mutant allele producing the non-functioning product, while in each affected male there is only the mutant allele with its non-functioning product and the Y chromosome, no normal gene product at all. Affected females are more prevalent in the general population because the female has two X chromosomes, either of which could carry the mutant allele, while the male only has one X chromosome as a target for the mutant allele. When the disease is no more deleterious in males than it is in females, females are about twice as likely to be affected as males. As shown in Pedigree Fig. 6.6, X-linked dominant inheritance has a unique heritability pattern.

The key for determining, whether a dominant trait is X-linked or autosomal is to look at the offspring of the mating of an affected male and a normal female. If the affected male has an affected son, then the disease is not X-linked. All of his daughters must also be affected if the disease is X-linked.

**Example**

## Hypophosphatemia

X-linked dominant inheritance is relatively rare. This disease is characterized by abnormally low levels of phosphorus in the blood due to defective re-absorption of phosphate in the kidneys. Calcium and Vitamin D metabolism are also abnormal resulting in softening of bones and rickets and this condition is called Vitamin D- resistant rickets.

### *c.ii. Sex Linked recessive inheritance*

Everyone has heard of some X-linked recessive disease even though they are, in general, rare. Hemophilia, Duchenne muscular dystrophy, Lesch-Nyhan syndrome are relatively rare in most populations, but because of advances in molecular genetics they receive attention in the media. More common traits, such as glucose-6-phosphate dehydrogenase deficiency or color blindness, may occur frequently enough in some populations to produce a few affected females. However, their effect on individuals is rarely life threatening and medical intervention is not needed.

The four features are:

1. As with any X-linked trait, the disease is never passed from father to son.
2. Males are much more likely to be affected than females. If affected males cannot reproduce, only males will be affected.
3. All affected males in a family are related through their mothers.
4. Trait or disease is typically passed from an affected grandfather, through his carrier daughters, to half of his grandsons.

**Table 6.2** X-linked recessive inheritance

| *Affected Father's Genotype* | | | | *Normal Father's Genotype* | | | |
|---|---|---|---|---|---|---|---|
| | | $X^A$ | Y | | | X | Y |
| Normal | X | $XX^A$ | XY | Carrier | $X^A$ | $X^AY$ | $X^AY$ |
| Mother's | | | | Mother's | | | |
| Genotype | X | $XX^A$ | XY | Genotype | X | XX | XY |
| All daughters carriers, all sons normal. | | | | Half of sons affected, half of daughters | | | |

In the Pedigree (Fig. 6.7), II-2 and II-5 are both carriers, their father was affected and passed on his only X chromosome to his daughters. II-3 cannot be a carrier for two reasons. First, males are either affected or normal, never carriers. Second, he didn't inherit his father's X chromosome. He inherited his father's Y chromosome. III-3 couldn't have been a carrier since neither her father nor her mother had the mutant gene.

**Example**

## Colour blindness, Hemophilia and Dushnne Muscular Dystrophy

(details in Chapter 10)

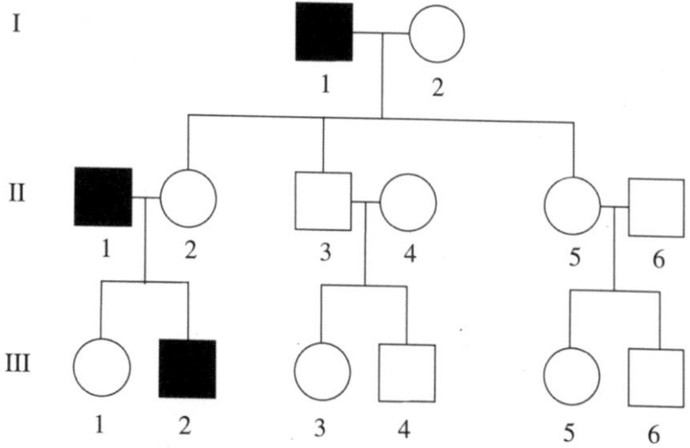


**Fig. 6.7** Pedigree for X-linked recessive inheritance

### *d. Y-Linked Inheritance*

Very few genes have been detected on the Y chromosome. In humans Y is less than half the length of the X chromosome.

The features are:

1. Trait expression and transmission is only in males, the individuals with the Y chromosome.
2. If a male has a trait, so should his father and paternal grandfather as well as his sons and their sons. It follows the inheritance of the Y chromosome.

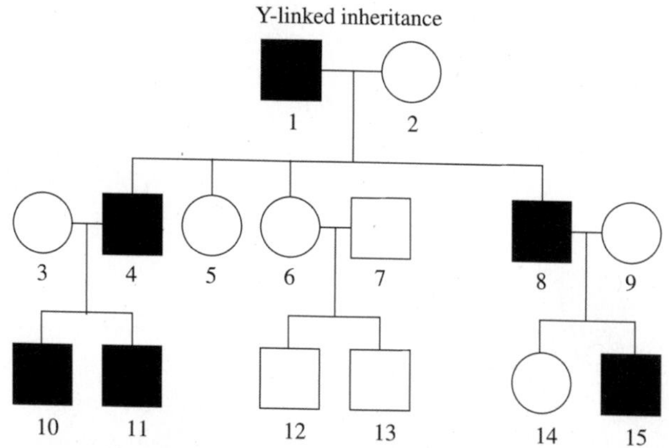


**Fig. 6.8** Pedigree for Y-linked inheritance

In the above pedigree all the male descendants of I-1 are affected. The sons III-12 and13 of II-7 are not affected since they carry the Y of their unaffected father II-7

**Example**

**Hairy pinna**, where there is excessive growth of hair in the external ear.

CHAPTER 7

# Human Chromosome Complement

## INTRODUCTION

In 1956 Joe-Hin Tjio and Albert Levan, working with specialized techniques established the exact number of human chromosomes in a human lung cell in a culture to be 46, three years after the discovery of DNA structure. The study of human cytogeneticists confirmed the study of Tjio and Levan in a variety of human cells in culture.

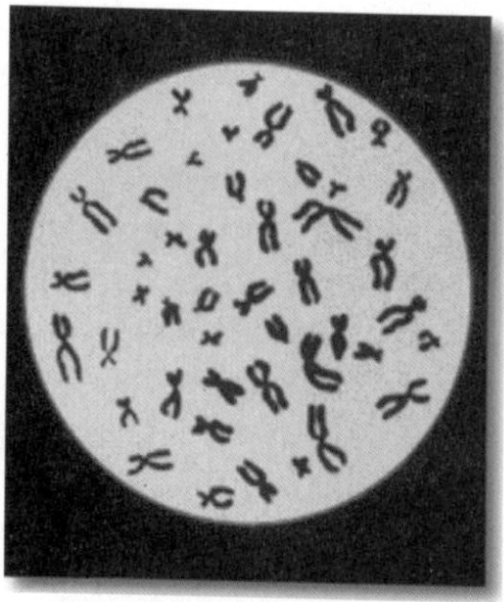

**Fig. 7.1** Human chromosome complement (Source: www.colarado.edu)

## 7.1 HUMAN CHROMOSOME PREPARATION

There are numerous methods available for preparing human chromosomes for study. Each has unique advantages and disadvantages. The chosen technique depends on the type of analysis undertaken. Individual chromosomes can usually be identified during cell division. Chromosomes in the metaphase and late prophase stages of cell division have the unique property of appearing as doublets. They can be distinguished by size, shape and the patterns produced by various stains. For study, human chromosomes are isolated from white blood cells and stimulated to divide in a culture medium with a mitogen (e.g. Phytohaemagglutinin) which increases the rate of cell division. Special treatment with the mitotic inhibitor for example colchicine stops cell division at metaphase stage, when chromosomes are clear and highly condensed. The cells are processed and dropped onto a micro slide, and air dried. The slides are then stained and photographed.

## 7.2 HUMAN KARYOTYPE

The chromosomes of a body cell occur in pairs. For any one chromosome of a particular size and shape, there is usually another match to it and are said to be homologous. When the chromosome set is inspected, it is seen that the length of the chromosome arms vary from one group of chromosomes to another. This is due to variation in the location of the centromere, the constricted region which holds the two arms together.

In some chromosomes the centromere is in the center, so that the two arms of the chromosomes are of equal length. Such a chromosome is called **metacentric** and the centromere is said to be median in position. If the centromere is slightly off the center, it is said to be submedian. The chromosome is then classified as **submetacentric** and will have one arm somewhat longer than the other. If the centromere is located at one end, then one arm is distinctly longer in relation to the other, which may appear tiny. The chromosome is then termed as **acrocentric**.

The chromosomes could be paired and systematically arranged according to the descending order of size and position of centromere and the systematic arrangement of chromosomes is termed a **karyotype**.

In human karyotype, 7 groups from A to G can be recognized. In the female every chromosome has a matching pair. But in a male one pair does not match. These are the sex chromosomes distinctly different in appearance, a large X and a small Y. All the chromosomes in a cell other then the sex chromosomes are called autosomes. The autosomes are numbered 1-22 on the basis of decreasing size. A human female thus has 22 pairs of autosomes plus two XX chromosomes. In contrast, a human male cell has 22 pairs of autosomes plus one X chromosome and one Y. On the basis of size, the X chromosome is placed in group C and Y in group G. Chromosomes are numbered based on their descending order of length. The largest chromosome has the lowest number i.e. 1 and the smallest chromosome the highest number i.e. 22.

Table 7.1 Classification of human chromosomes

| Group | Chromosome | Number Features |
|---|---|---|
| A | 1, 2, 3 | Large,metacentric |
| B | 4, 5 | Large, submetacentric |
| C | 6-12 & X | Medium size, submetacentric |
| D | 13, 14, 15 | Medium size, acrocentric |
| E | 16, 17, 18 | Shorter than group D; Metacentic or submetacentric |
| F | 19, 20 | Short, metacentric |
| G | 21, 22 &Y | Very short, acrocentric |

In addition to centromere, some chromosomes have a secondary constriction. For example the five pairs of chromosomes in D and G exhibit secondary constrictions near the tips of their short arms. These nucleolar organizer regions (NOR) give rise to nucleoli. The sites and number of NORs are constant for a given species. In human diploid cells there are ten. Group D and G chromosomes may also have tiny knob like structures called **satellites** at the very tips of their short arms. **Fragile sites** are non-staining gaps seen on several chromosomes. A common fragile site is often located in the q arm of the X chromosome and is clinically significant.

An individual's karyotype is often described with cytogenetic shorthand than by a picture. In a simplest form a normal human karyotype is described with their number and followed by the sex chromosomes. For example the normal female karyotype is indicated as 46, XX and that of a male as 46, XY.

Deviations from the normal karyotype may be associated with abnormalities. To describe abnormalities in chromosome structure and number, cytogeneticists use standardized symbols. For example a boy with typical Down syndrome is designated 47, XY, +21. He has 47 chromosomes and that extra chromosome is chromosome 21. The karyotype of a female with Turner syndrome is 45, X. This means that she lacks one X chromosome.

Diagonal lines indicate mosaicism. For example 46/47 designate the occurrence of two cell lines in the person, one with 46 chromosomes and the other with 47 chromosomes.

Abbreviations used

| | |
|---|---|
| del | deletion |
| dup | duplication |
| i | isochromosome |
| ins | insertion |
| inv | inversion |
| r | ring chromosome |
| s | satellite |
| t | translocation |

+ or – symbols, when placed before the chromosome number indicates an extra or loss of a whole chromosome. For example, +21 or –X. If these symbols are placed after chromosome number then

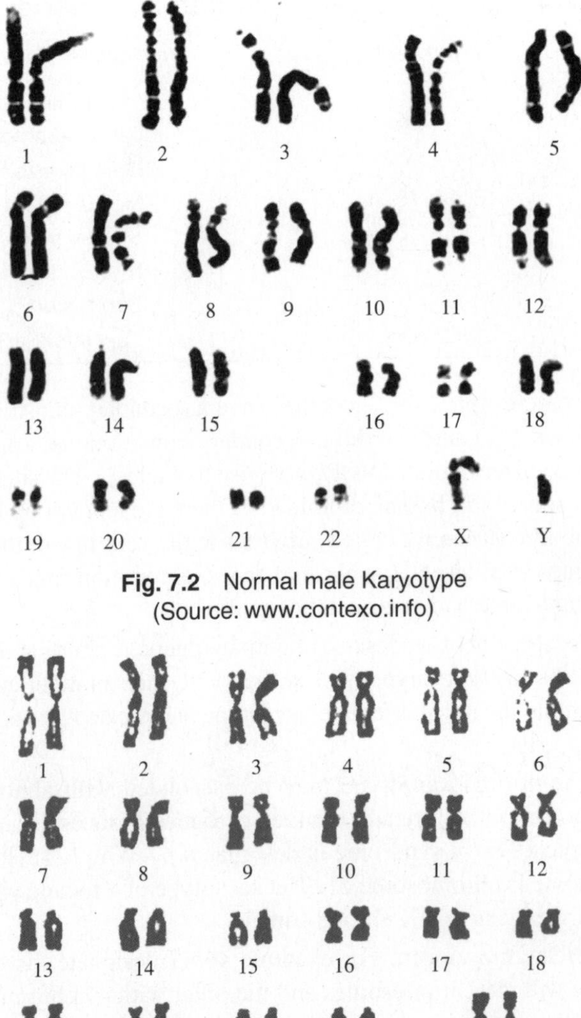

**Fig. 7.2** Normal male Karyotype
(Source: www.contexo.info)

**Fig. 7.3** Normal female Karyotype
(Source: www.contexo.info)

it indicates increase or decrease in the length of the chromosome. In the case of cri du chat syndrome the loss of the part of short arm of chromosome 5 is indicated as 5p-.

## Chromosome Banding

The traditional techniques used dyes that stain uniformly and produced uniform coloration in chromosomes. In 1970 Caspersson et al. introduced newer staining procedures and different dyes that produce dark and light cross bands of varying widths. Each chromosome in a haploid set has a unique banding pattern and now can be distinguished from other chromosomes of similar size and shape.

Generally there are four kinds of banding such as Giemsa or G banding, centromeric or C banding, Quniacrine or Q banding and Reverse or R banding.

### G Banding

This is widely used procedure. It involves Giemsa stain after trypsin treatment of metaphase chromosome to differentiate chromosome bands. When viewed under microscope the chromosomes show dark bands (G bands) and light bands (R bands). By this method approximately 400 dark and light bands could be resolved in a haploid set of chromosomes.

### C Banding

It requires heating in an alkali solution and staining with Giemsa. C bands are areas of consititutive heterochromatin located adjacent to the centromeres of all the chromosomes.

### Q Banding

This procedure uses Quinacrine mustard to stain chromosomes. They are observed under fluorescence microscopy. Bright Q bands are equivalent to G bands.

### R Banding

This is Reverse banding. It uses Giemsa under elevated temperature to produce the reverse pattern to that seen in G banding.

### AgNOR Staining

It is the silver staining of the nucleolus organizing (NOR) regions mark the ribosomal genes that are active in transcription. It is commonly seen on the D and G group of chromosomes.

### High Resolution Banding or Pro Metaphase Banding

In this technique DNA synthesis is arrested in a cell culture by methotrexate (folic acid antagonist) so that the cells are synchronized. The addition of folic acid removes the block. The culture is harvested by colchicines. Numerous cells are found to be in early metaphase before they become highly condensed. This reveals 800 or more bands per a haploid set.

### Flow Cytometry

The cells to be analyzed are ruptured and selectively stained with fluorescent dye for DNA. They are projected as a fine jet through a flow chamber across a laser beam which excites the chromosomes to fluoresce. This method is termed fluorescent activated cell sorter (FACS).

### Chromosome Features

The Paris conferences of 1971 and 1975 have given scheme to the accurate identification of parts of individual chromosome. Each chromosome has usually two arms held together at the centromere. The short arm is 'p' arm and the long arm is 'q' arm. Regions and bands are numbered from the centromere out. To identify a band in the chromosome, a sequence of 4 items are used namely chromosome number, arm, region and band number. For example 9q34 refers to chromosome 9, the long arm, region 3 and band 4.

## 7.3 CHROMOSOME PAINTING

In 1980s a technique **'FISH'** (fluorescent in situ hybridization) is developed to prepare brilliantly colored whole chromosomes. This technique requires complex mixtures of specially constructed DNA sequences called 'probes' that are complementary to different chromosome regions, together with a set of fluorescent dyes. Also needed are, a special microscope with special optical filter sets, as well as computer software to analyze the images and convert them into a dazzling multicolored display. Chromosome painting is useful for quickly detecting cells with extra or less chromosomes or with other structural abnormalities especially in the cancer cells.

Automated analysis is the recent development in the study of standard chromosome preparations. It involves methods of staining in cultures than on slides and having the chromosomes automatically sorted out and karyotyped by machines with special photometric and computer capabilities.

## 7.4 ARTIFICIAL CHROMOSOMES

In the early 1980s, scientists first produced tiny artificial chromosome in yeast. Human chromosomes are 100 times larger and much more complex than the Yeast artificial chromosome. But in 1997, Huntington Willard and his colleagues constructed human artificial microchromosomes from synthesized centromeric and telomeric DNA plus some genomic DNA. These tiny chromosomes are one-fifth to one-tenth the size of normal human chromosomes and could be replicated for six months (about 250 cell divisions) in the culture. These human microchromosomes can accept and express human genes, an important first step toward the possibility of treating certain genetic disorders by inserting normal genes into abnormal somatic cells. In addition they are valuable tool in the study of human chromosome structure.

CHAPTER 8

# Genetic basis of Sex

## INTRODUCTION

Sex is a character distinguished as maleness and femaleness. The egg producing individuals are females and sperm producing individuals are males. The sex is usually determined by a series of developmental changes under genetic and hormonal control. However, often one or a few genes can determine which pathway the development takes place.

Stevens (1905), Bridges (1922) and Goldschmidt (1938) found that chromosomes play a role in sex determination. The genes responsible for sex are located on the sex chromosomes, which are **heteromorphic** i.e. are morphologically dissimilar. X chromosome is medium in size and submetacentric i.e. the centromere is sub median in position and carries large amount of DNA. It belongs to 'C' group of chromosomes. On the other hand Y chromosome is small acrocentric i.e. the centromere is shifted to one end and has less DNA. It belongs to 'G' group of chromosomes in a human karyotype.

## 8.1 MECHANISM OF SEX DETERMINATION

In human beings sex is determined by XY- chromosomal mechanism. In this system females have 46 chromosomes arranged in 23 homologous, **homomorphic** (look similar) pairs. There are 22 pairs of autosomes (AA) and a pair of sexchromosomes, XX. Males have 22 homomorphic (AA) and one heteromorphic pair, referred as XY pair. During meiosis, females produce gametes that contain only the X chromosomes and all ova are similar, whereas males produce two kinds of gametes X bearing (50%) and Y bearing (50%). For this reason, females are referred to as **homogametic** and males as **heterogametic**.

Men and women have numerous anatomical and physiological differences, but at the chromosomal level there is just one.

- All (normal) eggs of a human female contain one X chromosome
- Sperm can contain either an X or a Y chromosome

Upon fertilization,

- an X sperm and an X egg = baby girl
- a Y sperm and an X egg = baby boy

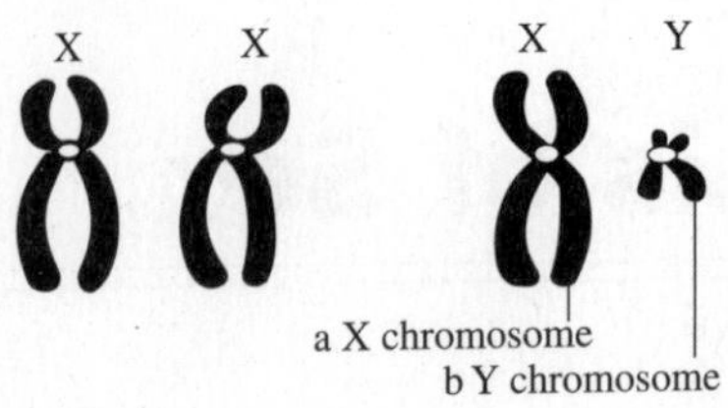


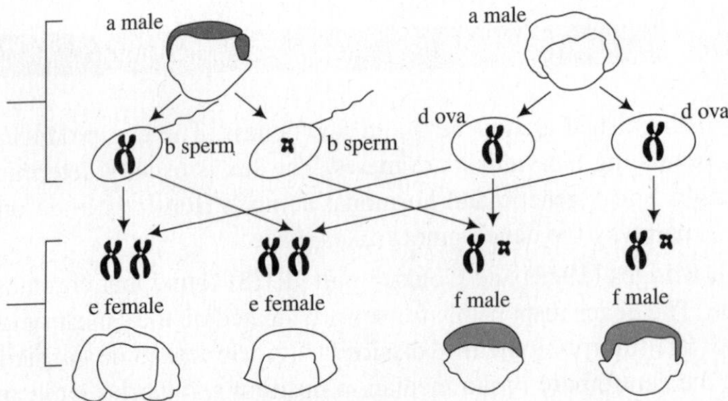


**Fig. 8.1** Sex determination mechanism
(Source: www.nature.com)

## Sex Determining Genes

Human embryologists had discovered that during the first month of embryonic development, the gonads that develop are neither testes nor ovaries. At about six or seven weeks of development, gonads become either ovaries or testes. For a long time, it was thought that a single gene, a testis – determining factor (**TDF**) located on the 'Y' chromosome acts as a sex switch to initiate male development.

Later it was found that males had a protein on their cell surfaces not found in females; this protein was called the **histocompatability Y antigen (H – Y antigen)**. The gene for this protein was found on the Y chromosome. This acted as sex switch, when present direct the gonad to develop into testis and when absent into ovaries.

In 1991, Robin Lovell-Badge and Peter Goodfellow isolated a gene called **sex-determining region Y (SRY)** lying adjacent to **ZFY gene** (Zinc finger on the Y chromosome). **ZFY gene** controls the initiation of sperm cell development. The gene **SRY** has been positively identified as the testis – determining factor because, when injected into normal (XX) female mice, it caused them to develop as males.

The Sry protein appears to bind at least two genes. One, the p450 aromatase gene, has a protein product that converts the male hormone testosterone to the female hormone estradiol; the Sry protein inhibits production of p450 aromatase. The second gene is the gene for Mullerian – inhibiting substance, which induces testicular development and the digression of female reproductive ducts; the Sry protein enhances this gene's activity. If the genes were absent, the gonads would develop into ovaries. Another gene is discovered and identified as the testis-determining factor.

Eva Eicher and Linda Washburn have developed a model in which two pathways of coordinated gene action help determine sex, one pathway for each sex. The first gene in the ovary – determining pathway is termed ovary determining (od) gene. The first gene in the testis – determining pathway must function before the od gene begins, in order to allow XY individuals to develop as males. Once the steps of a pathway are initiated, the other pathway is inhibited.

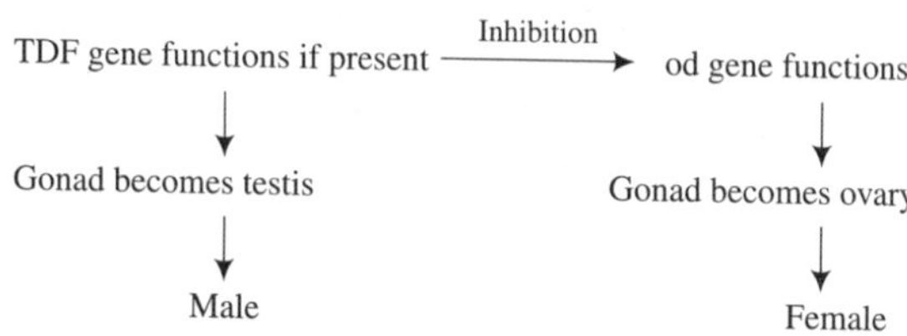


**Fig. 8.2** A Model for the initiation of gonad determination

## 8.2 DOSAGE COMPENSATION

In the XY chromosomal system of sex determination, males have only one X chromosome, whereas females have two. Males have half the number of X-linked alleles as females for genes which are not related to sex traits. In human beings and other mammals, the necessary dosage compensation is accomplished by the inactivation of one of the X chromosomes in females so that both males and females have only one functional X chromosome per cell.

### Lyon Hypothesis

In 1949 M. Barr and E. Bertram first observed a condensed body in the nucleus of the cells of a normal female cat and none in a male. They referred the body as **Barr body** or **Sex chromatin**. Mary Lyon then suggested that this Barr body represented an inactive X chromosome, which in females becomes tightly coiled into heterochromatin. This is called Lyon hypothesis. The number of Barr bodies is directly proportional to the extra X chromosomes. XO females have no Barr body. XX females have one and XXXX females have three. Females are considered sex chromatin positive and the human males are called sex chromatin negative. The sex chromatin is seen as a small darkly stained body with basic dyes in interphase cells. The frequency of its occurrence varies from tissues to tissues. In nervous tissue it may be 85%, in amniotic cells it is 95% and in oral smears it ranges from 20% to 25%. At the time of cell division one of the X chromosomes completes its replication of DNA later than the other, and is located peripherally, in the region of the nucleus where sex chromatin is found. The X chromosome which replicates late, condenses and separates from the rest and forms the sex chromatin.

In certain types of blood cells, like the polymorphonuclear leukocytes, the sex chromatin sticks out of the nucleus and consists of a head 1.5 m in diameter, connected to the nucleus by a filament called drumstick. The frequency of detectable drumsticks is low; 1 in 38 cells against 35 – 90 % for Barr bodies in other tissues.

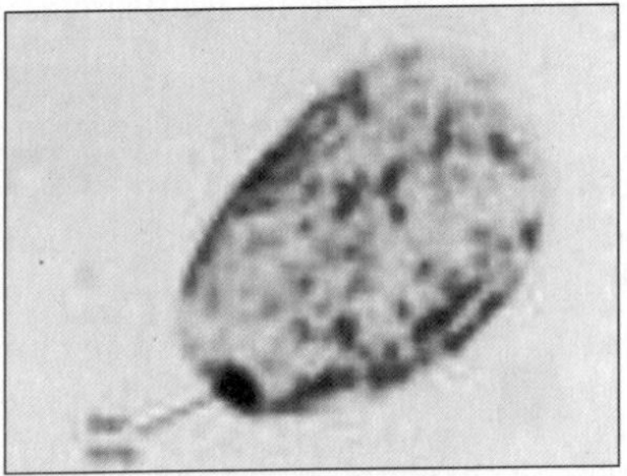

**Fig. 8.3** Barr body
(Source: www.britannica.com)

Genetic evidence supports Lyon hypothesis. Females heterozygous for a locus on the X chromosome show a unique pattern of phenotypic expression. In human females, one X chromosome is inactivated randomly in a cell. The inactive X can either be maternal or paternal in different cells of the same individual. Inactivation is random but once it has occurred, it remains fixed. The same X remains a Barr body for all future generations. Thus heterozygous females show **mosaiscism** at the cellular level for X-linked traits.

Glucose-6-phosphate dehydrogenase (G6PD) is an enzyme controlled by a gene in the X chromosome. The enzyme occurs in two forms A and B. Since they differ by an amino acid they can be distinguished by electrophoresis. The serum of a female heterozygote has both A and B forms, whereas any single cell has only one or the other, indicating that only one X is active in any particular cell.

The X chromosome is inactivated starting at a point called the X inactivation center (XIC). That region contains a gene called XIST (X inactive – specific transcripts). The XIST gene has been identified as the gene that initiated inactivation of the X chromosome. This gene is active only in the inactive X chromosome in a normal XX female. The gene product of XIST is an RNA that is not translated into a protein. It is found this RNA is associated with Barr bodies, coating the inactive chromosome.

## 8.3 SEX LIMITED GENES

The expression of sex involves the interaction of many genes with one another and with the environment. The genes determining maleness or femaleness are not only present in the sex chromosomes but also in the autosomes. Expression of sex and other characteristics depends upon the actions of an assortment of genes found in all the chromosomes.

Certain traits which are considered male or female are determined by genes carried by both sexes. For example, genes determining beard phenotype are not confined to the Y chromosome, even though the expression of the characteristic is normally confined to males. That genes on autosomes are involved is indicated by the fact that beard features found in father and his son may be very different. Genes that male receives from his mother can affect the beard growth. Therefore, a female must carry these genes which do not express themselves in her. Such genes whose expression is normally limited to just one of the sexes are called **sex-limited genes**. Their limited expression is due to the hormonal environment. Generally in the internal environment of both sexes, both male and female hormones are present. It is the proper balance of these hormones which determines the normal expression of certain genes. Genes for beard growth will act only when male hormone is present above a certain level. In some pathological conditions like a tumor in the adrenal cortex can cause excess secretion of androgens, the male hormones; as a consequence beard growth may occur in a female.

Breast development occurs only in a female but the genes for breast development occur in both the sexes. Genes for breast development depend on female hormone, estrogen which is secreted at a low level in males. Abnormal secretion of estrogen in male may cause breast development in male.

The role of hormones in triggering the expression of sex limited genes is evident in certain cases of precocious puberty, where sexual maturation takes place at a faster rate than in normal condition. Development of deep voice, which depends on male hormone, as well as other traits associated with masculine maturity, may be displayed by a boy who has not obtained maturity. This is caused often by the over secretion of the androgens. Precocious puberty may occur in a girl due to the excess secretion of estrogens. These conditions throw light on the influence of hormones over the expression of genes.

## 8.4 SEX INFLUENCED GENES

The sex influenced genes are present in the autosomes whose dominance is influenced by the sex of the bearer. These are expressed more frequently in one sex than in the other. In man premature baldness may occur due to disease, radiation or thyroid defects but, in some families baldness is found to be an inherited trait. In such inherited baldness, the hairs of a young man gradually become thin on head top, leaving ultimately a fringe of hairs low on the head, commonly known as pattern baldness is dominant in man and recessive in female. This is because the gene for baldness **(B)** in heterozygous state **(Bb)** expresses itself in male not in female. It means gene B for baldness behaves as a dominant in male and as a recessive in female.

| Genotype | Male | Female |
|---|---|---|
| BB | Bald | Bald |
| Bb | Bald | Not bald |
| Bb | Not bald | Not bald |

In man a nervous disease called Kuru has been found to be resulted by sex-influenced lethal genes. Individuals of both sexes homozygous for Kuru trait (K is dominant gene, k is recessive gene) die in childhood, usually before adolescence. Heterozygous (Kk) males act like carriers without any known effects, but heterozygous females die shortly after adolescence. The inheritance of gene for Kuru is as follows:

| Genotype | Male | Female |
|---|---|---|
| KK | Normal | Normal |
| Kk | Normal | Die after adolescence |
| kk | Die in childhood | Die in childhood |

CHAPTER 9

# Genetic Variation

## INTRODUCTION

Living organisms widely vary. Genes are responsible for similarities as well as dissimilarities between members of a family. Heritable variations are raw material for evolution. Without variations life will be monotonous. It is necessary to distinguish the inherited variation from that caused by the environment. If the source of variation is identified then the knowledge could be applied to such fields as human genetics, selective breeding and genetic engineering.

## 9.1 MUTATION

Inheritance is based on genes that are faithfully transmitted from parents to offspring during reproduction. Mechanisms have evolved to facilitate the faithful transmission of genetic information from generation to generation. Nevertheless "mistakes" or changes in the genetic material do occur. Such sudden, heritable changes in the genetic material are called mutations. An organism exhibiting a novel phenotype as a result of the mutation is termed mutant. The term "mutation" was introduced by Hugo De Vries. The mutation consisting of single changes in the nucleotide sequence is termed **'point mutation'**.

If the change is in the structure of a DNA molecule it is termed gene mutation and if it is in the structure or number of chromosomes in the cells of an organisms then it is termed as chromosomal mutation.

## Gene Mutation

Gene mutation is a change in the sequence of base pairs of a DNA molecule coding for a protein. There are four base pairs in a DNA. They are adenine, guanine, thymine and cytosine. The following could be the change in the base pairs:

- addition of one or more base pairs;
- deletion of one or more base pairs;
- substitution of one or more base pairs by others.

Often these changes in the DNA may alter the amino acids and affect the three dimensional structure of the protein. For example the change in the DNA triplet CTT to CAT alters the amino acid coded for from glutamic acid to valine. Such a change if it occurs in the beta globin chain of haemoglobin, results in sickle cell anemia.

Alteration in the reading frame of the triplet code of DNA (frame shift mutation) could be caused by either addition or deletion of a base pair. When a whole triplet of base pairs is deleted the polypeptide lacks one amino acid finally. Cystic fibrosis is the example for this kind, where 70% of the affected lack plenylalanine in the cell membrane. The deletion removes just one amino aid from a chain of 1480 amino aids.

A repetition of triplet base pairs may give rise to a string of similar amino acid in a polypeptide. It is called a **stutter** and is responsible for **Huntington's** disease where the triplet repeat inserts a series of glutamines in the polypeptide chain of the protein.

## Molecular basis of Gene Mutation

Though very accurate, the DNA replication some times shows inaccuracy which may occur within the DNA due to external or internal, natural or artificial factors. These introduce changes in the polynucleotide chain of a DNA molecule. The point mutations may be classified broadly into the following types:

1. Substitution mutations
2. Frame shift mutations

### *Substitution Mutations*

In a substitution mutation a nitrogenous base of triplet codon of DNA is replaced by another nitrogen base changing the codon. The altered codon may code for a different amino acid and may result in the formation of a protein molecule with a single amino acid substitution resulting in a altered phenotype. The substitution may be of the following two types.

#### a. Transitions

These are changes that involve replacement of one purine in a polynucleotide chain by another purine and correspondingly in the complementary chain the replacement of one pyrimidine by another pyrimidine.

The transitional substitutions can be introduced by any of the following ways either during DNA replication (**copy error mutation**) or otherwise.

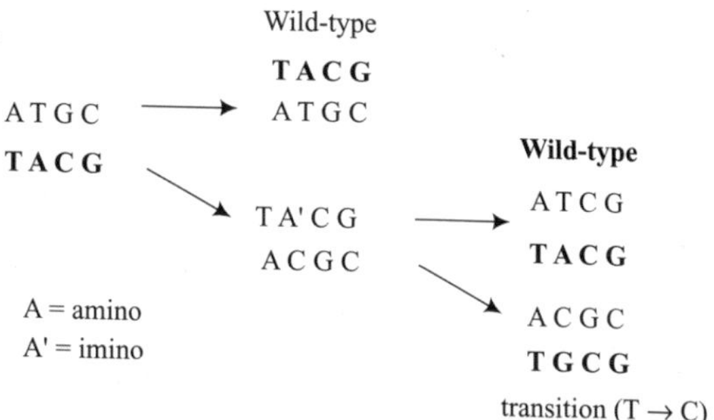


**Fig. 9.1** Transition mutation
(Source: www.mucn.ca)

## (i) Tautomerisation

In a normal DNA, the purine-adenine (A) is linked to the pyrimidine – thymine (T), by two bonds, while the purine – guanine (G) is linked to pyrimidine – cytosine (C) by three bonds. However, all these nitrogenous bases exist in alternate state. These states are called tautomers and are formed by the rearrangements in the distribution of hydrogen atoms (tautomeric shifts). Due to tautomerization the amino ($-NH_2$) group of cytosine and adenine is converted to imino (–NH) group and likewise keto group (C=O) of thymine and guanine is converted to end group (–OH).

In its tautomeric state, a nitrogenous base cannot pair with its normal partner. A tautomeric adenine pairs with normal cytosine and tautomeric guanine with thymine. Similarly tautomeric thymine pairs with normal guanine and cytosine with adenine. Such pairs of nitrogenous bases are known as "forbidden base pairs" or "unusual base pairs".

The rare bases can introduce mutations during DNA replication. For example, adenine in the parent DNA is in rare state, the complementary new chain will contain cytosine. At the time of next replication this cytosine would pair with guanine. This will produce a substitution of A = T base pair by G ≡ C pair. Similarly a situation of G ≡ C by A = T pair can be produced if cytosine is in tautomeric state.

## (ii) Ionization

Transitions may also be introduced by ionization of a base at the time of DNA replication. Ionization involves the loss of the hydrogen from number – 1nitrogen of a nitrogenous base. For example, in its ionized state, thymine pairs with normal guanine and ionized guanine links with normal thymine.

## (iii) Base analogs

Certain chemical compounds have molecular structure similar to the nitrogenous bases present in DNA nucleotides. These are called base analogs. There are usually derivatives of nitrogenous bases of DNA and occur as natural or artificial base analogs. Some of the natural base analogs are 5-methyl cytosine, 5-hydroxymethyl cytosine, 5-glucosyl hydroxymethyl cytosine, 5-hydroxymethyl uracil and 6-methyl purine. The artificial base analogs are 5-bromouracil (5 – BU), 5-iodouracil (5 – IU), 2 – bromo and 5 methyl-cytosine. The former two are base analogs of thymine and latter those of cytosine.

## 5 - Bromouracil

It is a structural analog of thymine. Its chemical structure is very much like that of thymine. It's keto form is more common while, the enol state is rare or it may occur in ionized state. Its normal keto form pairs with adenine and rare enol form pairs with guanine. When such mispairring (G = BU) occurs and DNA undergoes further replication, G pairs with C, while keto BU pairs with A which on further replication pairs with T. Thus G ≡ C pair is replaced by A = T base pair.

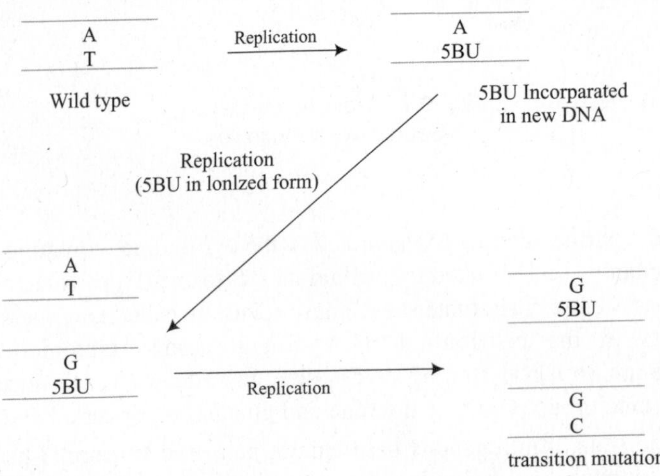


**Fig. 9.2** Copy error mutation (Source: www.answers.com)

## Aminopurine

It is a chemical artificial base analog of adenine. It can substitute adenine as well as can pair with cytosine.

### iv. Deamination

Certain chemical substances like nitrous acid, hydroxylamine, diethyl sulphate (DES), ethyl methane sulphate (EMS), ethyl ethane sulphate (EES), nitrosoguanidine (NTG) and nitrosomethyl urea (NMU) change the base sequence in DNA by series of chemical steps. Some of them like nitrous acid and hydroxylamine cause deamination of nitrogenous bases by replacing amino group by hydroxyl group. The deamination of cytosine leads to the formation of uracil, deamination of adenine forms hypoxanthine (H) and guanine forms Xanthine. Hypoxanthine exhibits bonding similarity with guanine.

At the time of DNA replication uracil pairs with adenine and hypoxanthine pairs with cytosine.This leads to the substitution of A = T for G ≡ C and G ≡ C for A = T.

## Transition Caused by Hydroxylamine

The hydroxylamine complexes with cytosine. This cytosine pairs with adenine rather than with guanine. This at the time of DNA replication introduces T = A at this level.

### b. Transversions

Certain alkylating agents like ethyl methane sulphate (EMS) and methyl methane sulphate (MMS) induce substitution by two ways.

(i) by substituting a purine for purine or pyrimidine for a pyrimidine (transition).

(ii) by substituting purine for pyrimidine or a pyrimidine for a purine (transversion) i.e. changes A = T to C ≡ G.

For causing transversions, these chemical alkylate the purine nitrogenous bases in the nitrogen at the seventh position in the guanine and adenine and finally lead to its separation from the DNA strand. This is known as **depurination**. Depurination leaves a gap at that point. At the time of replication, any of the four bases can possibly get inserted at this place in the complementary strand. If the nucleotide inserted contains a pyrimidine, it is transition and if purine then it is **transversion**. In the next cycle of DNA synthesis a DNA molecule is formed which contains the complete transversion.

## Oxidative Reactions

Reactive forms of oxygen (superoxide radicals, hydrogen peroxide and hydroxyl radicals) are produced in normal metabolism, by radiation, ozone, peroxides and certain drugs. These reactive forms of oxygen damage DNA and induce mutations by bringing about chemical changes in the DNA. For example, oxidation converts guanine into 8-oxy-7, 8-dihydrodexyguanine, which frequently mispairs with adenine instead of cytosine, causing a GC to TA transversion mutation.

## Frame Shift Mutations

A point mutation may consist of replacement, addition or deletion of a base. This kind of mutation is **frame shift** mutation. The addition or deletion of a base produces dangerous effect on the cell or organism because they change the reading frame of a gene from the site of mutation onward.

A frameshift mutation causes two problems. First, all the codons from the site of change onward will be different and thus yield a useless protein. Second, stop-signal information will be misread. One of the new codons may be a nonsense codon, it is no longer recognized as such because it is in a different reading frame and therefore, the translation process continues beyond the end of the gene.

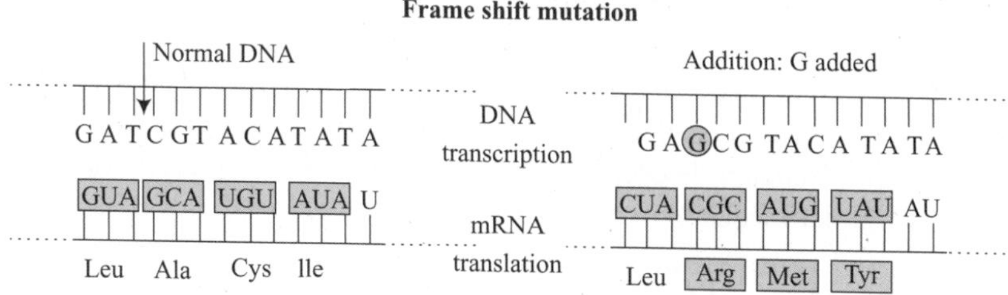


**Fig. 9.3** Frame shift mutation
(Source: www.staff.tushsd.kl2.az.us)

## Origin of Frame-shift Mutation

Acridine dyes cause deletion or insertion of a single base pair. Acridines like 5-aminoacridine and proflavin become intercalated between two adjacent purines and thus increase the distance between them from 3.4A° to 6.8A°. At the time of DNA replication, either a nitrogenous base pair is introduced in the gap or a nitrogenous base pair is lost.

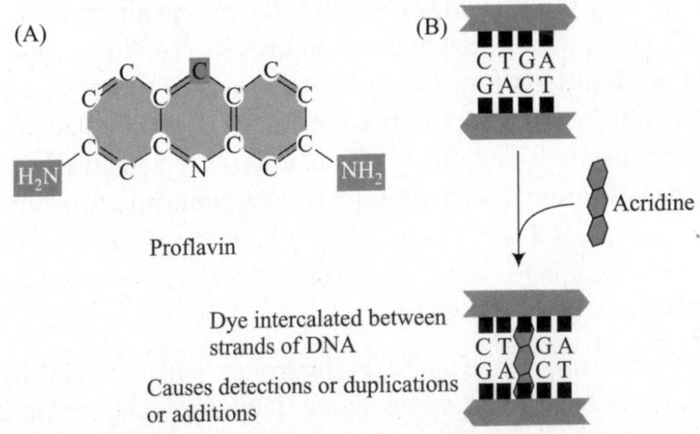


**Fig. 9.4** Mutation by intercalating agents (Source: www.academic.brooklyn.cuny.edu)

### *DNA repair*

If DNA replication proceeds normally, mutations would not occur. But replication is not always accurate. It is noted that out of every 10 billion base pairs is in error after a round of replication. The DNA polymerase enzyme removes the error normally. DNA polymerase has a proofreading function and thus minimizes the errors in replication of DNA. This is a repair function. In addition to errors in replication, DNA is subjected to the damaging effects of environmental agents such as UV rays. UV radiation strongly interacts with DNA and causes the formation of thymine dimers which distort the DNA molecule and interferes with replication. Normally the DNA is repaired by enzymes that recognize the distortion, bind to the damaged region, and either remove the dimer or split it. If the dimer is removed, DNA polymerase fills in the gap, with the help of DNA ligase. If the dimer is not removed, an error-prone repair system enables the insertion of incorrect bases opposite the dimer. This process causes high mutation rate.

Since the repair of damaged DNA is controlled by enzymes, and since enzymes are coded by genes, it is evident that mutations can affect the repair function. The recessive disease **xeroderma pigmentosum** (XP) is an example of a malfunctioning repair process. In this condition there is failure of DNA repair mechanism. People with xeroderma pigmentosum are extremely sensitive to sunlight and have a high incidence of skin cancer.

The three autosomal recessive diseases namely Bloom's syndrome (BS), Fanconi's anemia (FA) and Ataxia telangiectasia (AT) there is chromosomal instability and the chromosomes break often. In all these three conditions there is a high risk of cancer. In FA cells there is a defect in excising and repairing DNA damage; in BS cells, the rate of DNA replication is severely retarded.

## 9.2 MUTAGENS

Mutagens are agents, physical, chemical and biological causing mutations. There are two main classes of mutagens responsible for inducing mutations. They are (i) Radiation (ii) Chemicals.

### *(i) Radiation*

All forms of energy radiations that are capable of disrupting the chemical structure of genes have been found to be mutagenic. These include UV rays, X-rays, alpha rays, gamma rays and beta rays.

People are routinely exposed to low levels of radiation from cosmic, medical and environmental sources, but there have been natural and man made disasters that produced higher degree of radiation. Most data on human radiation exposure come from the study on atomic bomb explosion in 1945 in Hiroshima and Nagasaki. In 1986 The Chernobyl nuclear power plant in northern Ukraine exploded emitting high radiation. The Techa River in southern Russia is another place where people have been tragically exposed to higher amount of radiation. The neighbouring nuclear power plant dumped the nuclear sludge of plutonium into the Techa river exposing the inhabitants to a high degree of radiation.

### Biological effects

#### *1. Effect of ionizing radiations*

The ionizing radiations include X-rays, gamma rays, alpha rays, beta rays, neutrons and protons. The alpha and beta rays do not penetrate beyond the human skin, and therefore, do not affect body cells.

The gamma and X-rays collide with the molecules of the cells at high speed and eject electrons from the outer shells of atoms. The atoms therefore, become positively charged. In addition, the ejected electrons move at high speed and, in turn, knock other electrons free from their respective atom. When energy is dissipated, the free electrons attach to other atoms which then become negatively charged ions. These ions then undergo chemical reactions producing mutagenic effects.

These radiations produce breaks in the chromosomes and chromatids and abnormal mitosis in cells. The chromosome breaks leads into loss of chromosome segments, interchanging of segments and loss of genes.

#### *2. Effect of non-ionizing radiations*

Ultraviolet rays, have longer wave lengths and carry much more lower energy. The UV rays are absorbed by nucleic acids and cause alterations in the bond characteristics of purines and pyrimidines. The bases so altered are called **photoproducts**. Pyrimidines are more prone to such changes. Two adjacent pyrimidines of the same DNA strand are found to form covalent bonds forming **dimers**. This dimerization interferes with the proper base pairing of thymine with adenine and may result in the pairing of thymine with guanine. This results in base substitution.

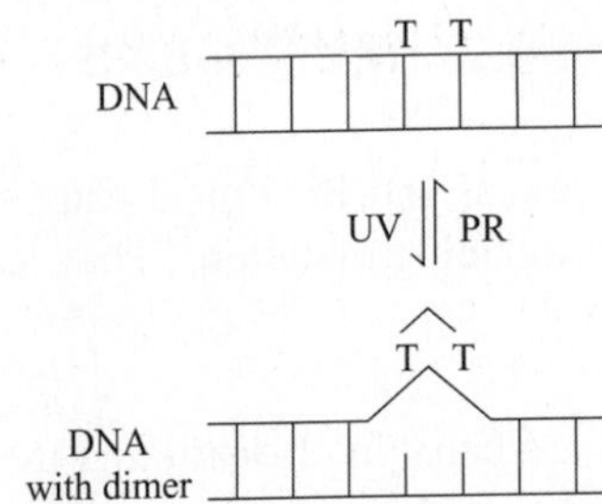


**Fig. 9.5** Dimerization by UV rays
(Source: www.dl.clackamas.edu)

### *(ii) Chemical mutagens*

The possible sources of chemical mutagens are unlimited. The list of chemical mutagens becomes longer with every passing year. Some of the most powerful mutagens are mustard gas, formaldehyde, ethylurethane, organic peroxides, acridine dyes, nitrous acid, 5-bromouracil and L.S.D. (lyseric acid dimethylamide).

The alterations that are caused by chemicals are already discussed in the earlier part of the chapter.

## 9.3 DETECTION OF MUTATION

Humans are exposed to a large number of chemicals in their daily lives. Most of them have mutation causing potential. It is vital that these chemicals are screened for their mutagenic nature before being put into use.

A simple test to detect mutations was introduced in 1974 by Bruce Ames and termed Ames test. It is based on the principle that result from damage to DNA. The Ames test uses four strains of the bacterium Salmonella typhimurium that have defects in the lipopolysaccharide coat, that normally protects the bacteria from chemicals in the environment. In addition, their DNA repair system is inactivated, making them susceptible to mutagens.

One of the four strains used in this can detect base-pair substitutions; the other three can detect frame shift mutations. Each strain carries a mutation his that renders them unable to synthesize the amino acid histidine, and the bacteria are plated on to medium that lacks histidine. Only bacteria that have undergone a reverse mutation of the histidine gene are able to synthesize histidine and grow on the medium. Chemicals that are to be tested for their mutagenic or carcinogenic capacity are added to plates inoculated with the bacteria, and the number of mutant colonies that appear on the plate are counted. The number of colonies that appear on control plates with no chemical are compared with the experimental plates with chemicals. Any chemical that significantly increases the number of mutant colonies on a treated plate is mutagenic and probably also carcinogenic. In 1975 a study was made in US to test the compounds in the hair dye sold in the market for mutagenic capacity using Ames test. It was proved that hair dye contained compounds that were mutagenic and then were removed from the hair dye.

## 9.4 CHROMOSOMAL VARIATIONS

Each species of animals or plants has a fixed number of chromosomes. These chromosomes are represented in haploid gametes and twice in diploid body cells. Sometimes changes occur in the structure or number of the chromosomes. These bring in major alterations in the cells or organisms. There are two major chromosomal alterations. They are associated with (i) Structure of the chromosomes (ii) Number of the chromosomes.

### *a. Chromosomal mutations*

There are visible changes in the structure of chromosomes, involving changes either in the total number of genes or gene loci in a chromosome or their rearrangement. These are also known as **chromosomal aberrations**. These arise from breaks in chromosomes and may be of the following four types:

A. Changes involving the number of gene loci
   1. Deficiency or Deletion
   2. Duplication or Addition

B. Changes involving the arrangement of gene loci
   3. Translocation
   4. Inversion

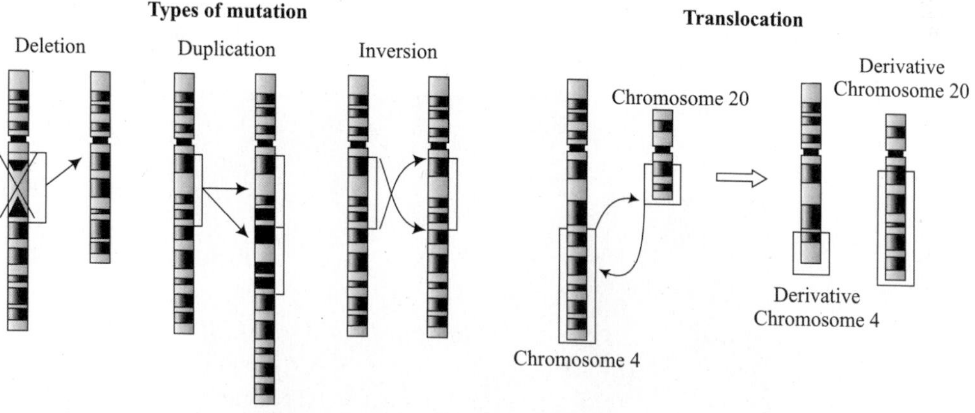


**Fig. 9.6** Types of chromosomal aberrations (Source: www.content.answers.com)

### *i. Deletion*

The deficiency is the deletion of a chromosomal segment resulting in the loss of genes. Depending on the length of the lost segment, the genes lost may vary from a single gene to a block containing many genes. A chromosome with segments ABCDEFGHIJ undergoes a deletion of segment C that would generate the mutated chromosome ABDEFGHIJ.

The break in the chromosome may be caused by several agents such as chemicals, radiations and viruses. The break occurs at random either in both the chromatids of a chromosome (chromosome break) or only in one chromatid (chromatid break).

The segment that is deleted does not survive, since it lacks the centromere. The portion of the chromosome carrying the centromere functions as genetically deficient chromosome.

## Types

Deletion may be of two types:

(a) **Terminal deletion:** It refers to the loss of segment from one or the other end of the chromosome. The terminal part fails to survive and causes terminal deletion. It is caused by a single break in the chromosome.

(b) **Intercalary deletion or Interstitial deletion:** It involves two breaks and an intermediate segment is deleted followed by the reunion of the terminal segments.

When an intercalary part of a chromosome is missing, a **buckling effect** (looping) may be observed microscopically, and this buckle like projection is formed by the normal part of the chromosome which corresponds to the missing part of the deletion chromosome.

In humans, a deletion in the short arm of chromosome 5 is responsible for **cri-du-chat** syndrome. The name derives from the peculiar, cat-like cry of infants with this syndrome. A child with this syndrome has a small head, widely spaced eyes, a round face, and mental retardation.

Since deletions involve loss of genetic material, these have some deleterious effect on the organism and is dependent upon the amount and quality of genetic material lost. A deletion might be small without producing any detectable change in the organism. But the deletions of large size

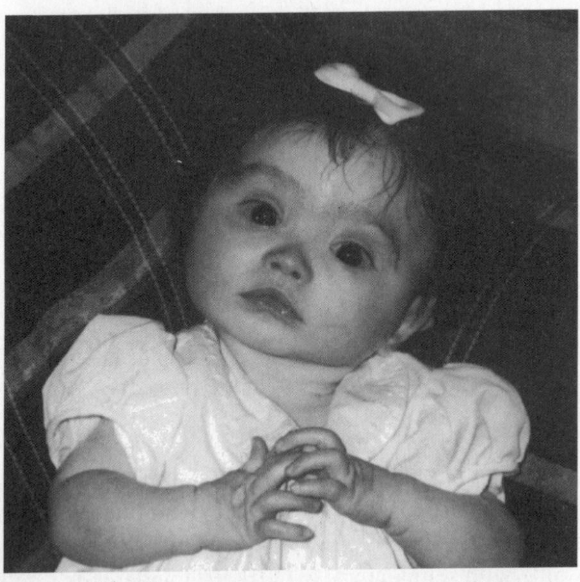

**Fig. 9.7** A Baby with Cri du chat syndrome
(Source: www.criduchat.u-net.com)

are lethal to the organisms. Deletions may allow recessive mutations on the undeleted chromosome to be expressed. This phenomenon is referred to as **pseudodominance**.

### *ii. Duplication*

The presence of same block of genes more than once in a haploid complement is known as **duplication** and the additional segment is called a repeat. In a chromosome with segments ABCDEFG, duplication may include once DE segments giving rise to an abnormal chromosome with segments ABCDEDEFG or thrice resulting in ABCDEDEDEFG.

#### Types

Three types of duplication have been recognized:

(a) **Tandem duplication:** In this duplication the added segment has the same genetic sequence as is present in the original state in the chromosome. For example, if duplication piece is ABC, tandem duplication will be ABCABCDEF.

(b) **Reverse tandem duplication:** In such duplication the sequence of genes aligned in the attached chromosome piece is just the reverse of the original segment. For example, if duplicated piece is ABC, the reverse tandem will be ABCCBADEF.

(c) **Displaced duplication:** In displaced duplication the chromosomal segment gets located some distance from the original segment, either on the same chromosome or on a different one. An example for this is ABCDEFGDE.

An example of duplication in Drosophila is the **Bar eye**. The gene for Bar eye is located in the 16A region of the X chromosome. In homozygous Bar eye there are two 16A regions. In heterozygous double bar the 16A is represented in three times and the effect is severe.

In humans, duplications are observed on 4$^{th}$ chromosome, resulting in infants with small head, sloping forehead, hand abnormalities and mental retardation.

### Significance

Duplications are more frequent and less deleterious. These do not lower the viability, but do produce abnormality of structure and function. In chromosome pairing problem arises at prophase I of meiosis, because the two chromosomes are not homologous throughout their length.

Duplication play significant role in evolution, because duplication increases number of genes in the chromosome complement.

### *iii. Translocation*

Translocation is a kind of chromosomal rearrangement in which a block of genes from one non-homologous chromosome is transferred to another non-homologous chromosome. Translocation should not be confused with crossing over, in which there is exchange of genetic material between homologous chromosomes.

If a chromosome has AB genes and another chromosome CD and exchange of genes result in exchange segment AD and CB, this is translocation.

Types

(a) **Non-reciprocal translocation:** Here the genetic material moves from one chromosome to another without any reciprocal exchange. For example, in the following two non-homologous chromosomes the gene arrangement is ABCDEFGHIJ and KLMNOPQ. If chromosome segment EF moves from the first chromosome to the second without transfer of segment from the second chromosome to the first, a non-reciprocal translocation has taken place producing chromosomes ABCDGHIJ and KLMNOPEFQ.

(b) **Reciprocal translocation:** It is the exchange of parts between non homologous chromosomes. It is produced by single break in each of the two non homologous chromosomes and exchange of parts. A reciprocal translocation between the two chromosomes might give rise to chromosomes QEFGHIJ and KLMNOPDCBA.

(c) **Robertsonian translocation:** In this type, the long arms of two acrocentric chromosomes become joined to a common centromere through a translocation, generating a metacentric chromosome with two long arms and another chromosome with two very short arms. The small chromosome fails to segregate, leading to an overall reduction in the number of chromosomes. Robertsonian translocation is the cause of some cases of Down syndrome.

## Effects of Translocation

During synapsis in cell division, pairing of translocated chromosome takes up a "cross-shaped" configuration. Translocations result in new linkage arrangements, position effects and semi-sterility.

In a reciprocal translocation heterozygote (the two normal and two translocated) chromosomes pair to form a cross-shaped configuration at pachytene of meiosis, whereas the normal chromosomes form a bivalent. The occurrence of crossing over and chiasmata formation in each arm, results in the formation of a ring or circle of four chromosomes at the diakinesis and at the metaphase of first meiotic division.

The anaphasic movement of chromosomes towards the poles takes place in any one of the three different ways given below.

(i) **Alternate segregation:** The alternate chromosomes of the ring go to the same pole; the normal chromosomes on one pole and the translocated chromosomes on the other pole. Therefore, all the gametes receive full complement and are fully viable.

(ii) **Adjacent – 1 – segregation:** In open ring configuration, one normal and one translocated chromosome reach one pole and one translocated and one normal chromosome to the other pole. Here, both types of gametes are unbalanced, carrying duplications and deletions that are usually lethal.

(iii) **Adjacent-2-regregation:** In some translocations, the two chromosomes (one normal and other translocated) go to one pole and the other two go to the other pole. So, four types of gametes are formed.

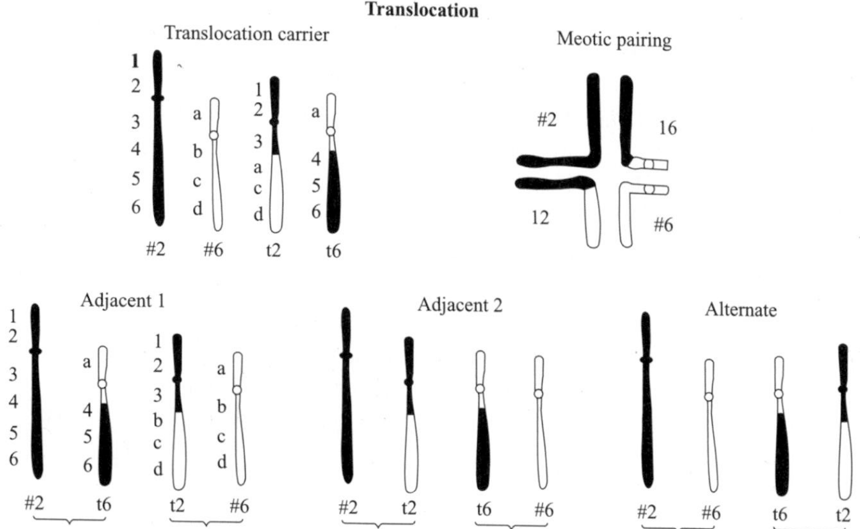


**Fig. 9.8** Effects of translocation
(Source: www.usd.edu)

**Example**

**Philadelphia Chromosome**

The Philadelphia chromosome is produced by translocation of the long arm of 22nd chromosome and the long arm of chromosome no. 9. This results in chronic myeloid leukemia. At the end of a normal chromosome 9 is a potential cancer causing gene called abl. As a result of the translocation, a part of the abl gene is fused with the bcr gene from chromosome 22. The protein produced by this fusion gene abl-bcr is much more active than the protein produced by the normal abl gene; the fusion protein increases the unregulated cell division and eventually leads to leukemia.

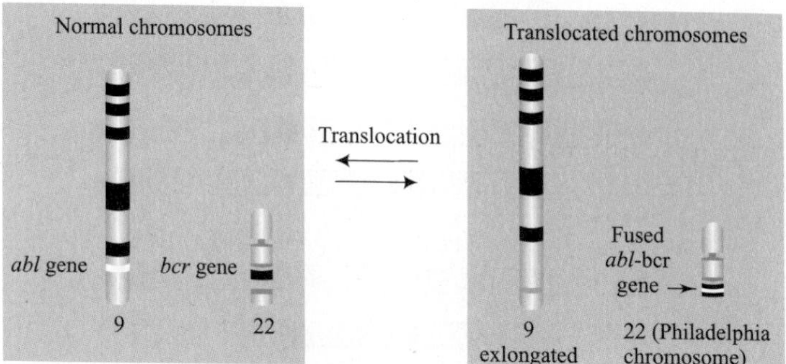


**Fig. 9.9** Philadelphia chromosome
(Source: www.cardynshope.com)

## Significance

(i) Translocation may cause change in the morphology or appearance of chromosomes by centric fusion between two acrocentric chromosome segments. This may lead to the change in the number of chromosomes.

(ii) Translocation introduces genetic polymorphism in the populations and plays a role in formation of new species.

(iii) Translocation may play an important role in the evolution of animals. For example Chimpanzees, Gorillas and Orangutan have 48 chromosomes and humans have 46. The G-banding pattern of the 2nd chromosome, a large metacentric chromosome in man matches with two acrocentric chromosomes in apes. A robertsonian translocation would have given rise to human in evolution from apes, by reduction in the number of chromosome.

### *iv. Inversion*

Sometimes the number of genes in a chromosome is not changed but the sequence of genes is altered by the rotation of gene segment within a chromosome by 180°. For example if a chromosome having gene sequence ABCDEFGHIJ breaks and the middle segment CDEF undergoes inversion; the gene sequence in the inverted chromosome will be ABFEDCGHIJ.

Types

(a) **Paracentric inversion:** When both the breaks in the chromosome during inversion occur on the same side of the centromere, the inversion is known as **paracentric**. The inverted segment is without a centromere. For example ABFEDCG . HIJ is paracentric inversion as depicted in the figure. If paracentric inversion occurs singly, i.e. on one side of the centromere alone, it is known as intraradial or homobrachial. On the otherhand, when two paracentric inversions occur one on either side of the centromere, the inversion is known as interradial or brachial inversion.

(b) **Pericentric inversion:** In **pericentric** inversion the inverted segment contains the centromere i.e. it involves one break on either side of the centromere. For example, as given in figure, ABCH . GEFDIJ

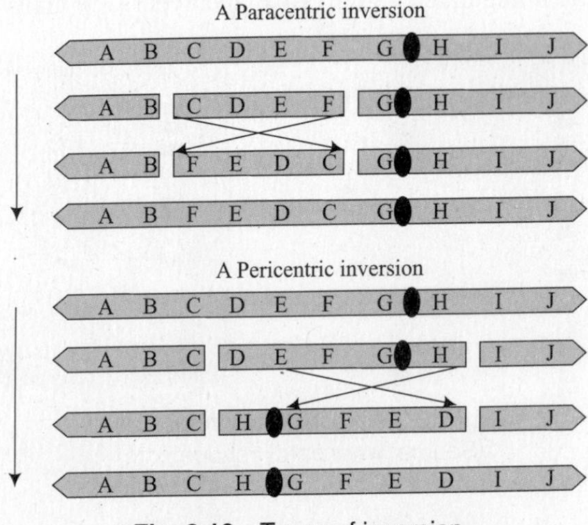


**Fig. 9.10** Types of inversion
(Source : www.depts.washington.edu)

### Effects

At the time of gamete formation, inversion disrupts pairing and abnormal configurations are obtained. The paracentric inversion with one chiasmata in the region of inversion, results in the formation of an **acentric** chromatid lacking centromere, and a **dicentric** chromatid connecting the two chromosomes. The acentric and dicentic chromatids are inviable. Because of the dicentric chromosome in anaphase I of meiosis, the centromeres are pulled toward opposite poles by a dicentric bridge which finally breaks.

Crossing over in a pericentric inversion results in the formation of the chromosomes which have duplications for certain genes and deletion for others. Pericentric inversion changes the appearance of a chromosome. A chromosome with median centromere ('V' shaped), may change into hook-shaped or rod-shaped form.

Effects of inversion on phenotype may be the occurrence of **position effect**. A gene in one location on a chromosome does not necessarily have the same action that it could have in another position.

Inversions suppress crossing over and tend to retain the original combination of genes.

Inversions help in the origin of new species. As a result of inversions the crossing over frequency is reduced and so recombination is less.

## Fragile Sites

Chromosomes sometimes develop constrictions or gaps at particular locations called fragile sites because they are prone to breakage under certain conditions. A number of fragile sites have been identified in human chromosomes. One of the common fragile sites is located in the X chromosome. It shows X linked inheritance and has several repeats of the sequence CGG.

Fragile X syndrome (FXS), is the most common cause of *inherited* mental impairment. This impairment can range from learning disabilities to more severe cognitive or intellectual disabilities (Sometimes referred to as mental retardation). FXS is the most common cause of autism or "autistic-like" behaviors. Symptoms also can include characteristic physical and behavioral features and delays in speech and language development.

Fragile X associated tremor ataxia syndrome (FTAS), a condition which affects balance, tremor and memory in some older male gene carriers.

Fragile X-related premature ovarian failure (POF), is a problem with ovarian function which can lead to infertility and early menopause in some female gene carriers.

### b. Variations in chromosome number

Chromosome mutation also includes change in the number of chromosomes. Anomalies of chromosome number occur as either **euploidy** or **aneuploidy**. Euploidy involves changes in whole sets of chromosomes; aneuploidy involves changes in chromosome number of addition or deletion of less than a whole set.

#### 1. Aneuploidy

There are four common types of aneuploidy:

(a) **Nullisomy** is the loss of both members of a homologous pair of chromosomes. It is represented as 2n-2, where n refers to the haploid number of chromosomes. Thus, among humans, a nullisomic person has 44 chromosomes.

(b) **Monosomy** is the loss of single chromosome represented as 2n – 1. A monosomic person has 45 chromosomes.

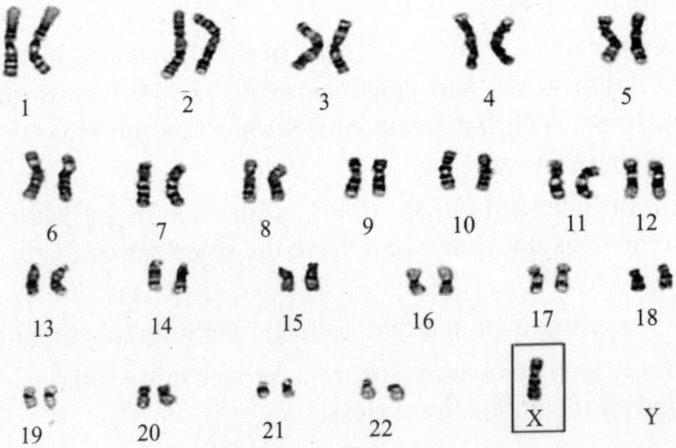

**Fig. 9.11** Monosomy
(Source: www.answers.com)

(c) **Trisomy** is the addition of a chromosome, a diploid cell with an extra chromosome is **trisomic** 2n + 1. A trisomic person has 47 chromosomes and there are three homologous copies of one chromosome.

(d) **Tetrasomy** is the gain of two homologous chromosomes, represented as 2n + 2. A tetrasomic person has 48 chromosomes.

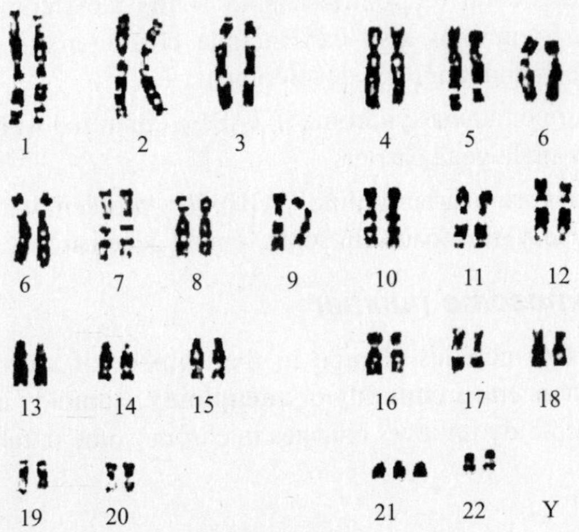


**Fig. 9.12** Trisomy
(Source: www.answers.com)

An individual that has an extra copy of two different (non homologous) chromosomes is referred to as double trisomic and represented as 2n+1+1. Similarly a double monosomic is represented as 2n-1-1 and a double tetrasomic as 2n+2+2.

Aneuploidy may result from non disjunction, the failure of homologous chromosomes or sister chromatids to separate in meiosis or mitosis. There is unequal separation of chromosomes between daughter cells during cell division. Non disjunction leads to some gametes or cells that contain an extra chromosome and others that are missing a chromosome.

The frequency of non disjunction is quite high in humans, but the results are usually so devastating to the growing zygote that miscarriage occurs very early in the pregnancy. If the individual survives, he or she usually has a set of symptoms - a syndrome -caused by the abnormal dose of each gene product from that chromosome.

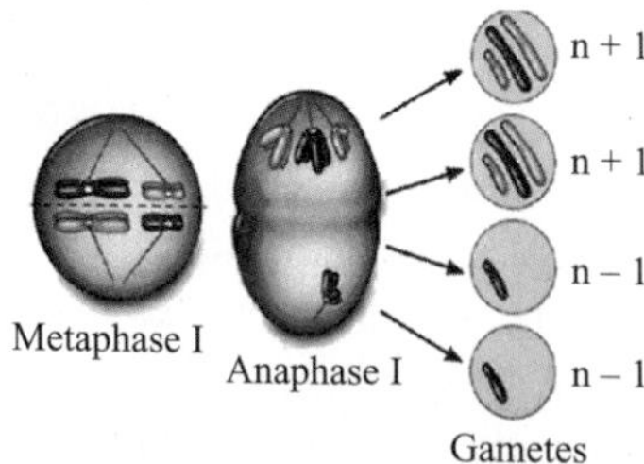


**Fig. 9.13** Non disjunction
(Source: www.ccs.k12.in.us)

Secondly aneuploidy may be caused by chromosomal lagging whereby one chromosome moves (laggard chromosome) more slowly than others during anaphase, is excluded from the telophase nucleus and thus is lost. The small chromosome created by Robertsonian translocation may be lost in mitosis or meiosis.

### 2. Mosaicism

Rarely, an individual is made up of several cell lines, each with different chromosome numbers. These individuals are referred to as **mosaics** or **chimeras**, depending on the sources of the cell lines. Such conditions can be the result of non-disjunction or chromosomal lagging during mitosis in the zygote or in nuclei of the early embryo. A lagging X chromosome is lost in one of the dividing somatic cells, resulting in an XX cell line and an XO cell line. In Drosophila, if this chromosomal lagging occurs early in development, an organism that is part male (XO) and part female (XX) develops. This may result in a fly half male and half female. A mosaic of this type with male and female phenotypes is termed **gynandromorph**.

Many sex chromosomal mosaics are known in humans, including XX / X, XY / X, XX / XY and XXX / X.

### 3. Aneuploids in Humans

The most common aneuploids seen in living humans are sex-chromosomal aneuploids. Turner syndrome and Kleinfelter syndrome are the examples.

Autosomal aneuploids are often spontaneously aborted early in development. The common autosomal aneuploid is trisomy 21, also called Down syndrome.

## Down Syndrome or Mongolism (47, XX or XY)

It was first reported by Langdon Down (1866). The defect is caused by trisomy of $21^{st}$ chromosome. The small extra chromosome is formed due to non disjunctional error during the formation of gametes where the $21^{st}$ chromosomes failed to separate. Most children with Down syndrome are born to normal parents. In most cases it arise from maternal nondisjunction and the frequency of this occurring correlates with maternal age. The occurrence of trisomy in live births and in spontaneous abortions increases with the age of the mother. Researches indicate that a mother of 35 years has more risk carrying a child affected by Down syndrome. The risk is 3% higher compare to mother of 25 years.

Down syndrome also occurs due to translocation of chromosomes 21 and 14 or 15. Since the facial features resembles that of a mongoloid race Down syndrome is also termed Mongolism.

The features are moon face, open mouth, projecting lower-lip, long-rigid tongue, stubby hands and feet, occurrence of simian line in the palm, slanting eyes, broad forehead, congenital malformations especially of the heart, low level of calcium in blood and susceptibility to respiratory orders. Mental retardation is observed and IQ is 25-50 compared with an average IQ of 100 in general population. Incidence is about 1/700 live birth.

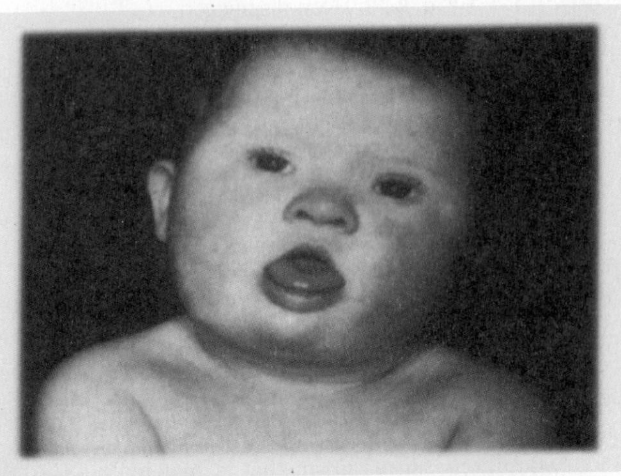

**Fig. 9.14** Down syndrome baby
(Source : www.manbir.online.com)

**Trisomy 18,** also known as **Edward syndrome,** arises with a frequency of approximately 1 in 8000 live births. Babies with Edward syndrome are severely retarded and have low set ears, a short neck, deformed feet, clenched fingers, heart problems and other disabilities. Few live for more than a year after birth.

**Trisomy 13** has a frequency of about 1 in 15,000 live births and produces features that are collectively known as **Patau syndrome**. Characteristics include severe mental retardation, a small head, sloping forehead, small eyes, cleft lip and palate, extra fingers and toes and numerous other problems. About half of children with Trisomy 13 die within the first month of life, and 95% die by the age of 3.

**Trisomy 8** is rarer and arises with a frequency of about 1 in 25,000 to 50,000 live births. This aneuploid is characterized by mental retardation, contracted fingers and toes, low set malformed ears, and a prominent forehead. Many who have this condition have normal life expectancy.

## Klinefelter Syndrome (47, XXY)

The male has one extra X chromosome, thus inhibiting the development of male characters. When an abnormal egg with XX chromosome is fertilized by a sperm carrying Y chromosome, a zygote with normal autosomes and XXY chromosomes is formed. Features are long legs, mental retardation, external genitalia are of male type but the testes are very small, body hair is sparse, feminized secondary sexual characters, female like breast development (gynecomastia) and no sperm production. They are infertile. Incidence is about 1/500 male births.

This condition can be treated by surgical removal of breast. Although sterility is unalterable, treatment with testosterone does promote development of sex organs, body hair, musculature and deeper voice.

## Turner Syndrome (45, XO)

The female lacks one X chromosome. This is produced when an egg with X chromosome is fertilized by a sperm without a sex chromosome. They are characterized by short stature, webbed neck, low set ears, hypoplastic nails, under-developed breast and broad shield like chest with widely spaced nipples, no ovary, uterus and no mensuration, hormonal abnormality, sexual hairs scanty, deformed heart, horse shoe shaped kidneys, double ureters and mental retardation. Additional skeletal deformities are seen sometimes: a high, arched palate, receding chin, mismatching of the upper and lower teeth and abnormally low bone density. They are sterile with gonadal dysgenesis (rudimentary gonad). Incidence is about 1/5000 female birth. It is highly lethal in embryos, being the most common type among spontaneous abortions and account for 20% of all chromosomally abnormal aborted embryos. 98% of Turner syndrome is lost during the first three months of pregnancy.

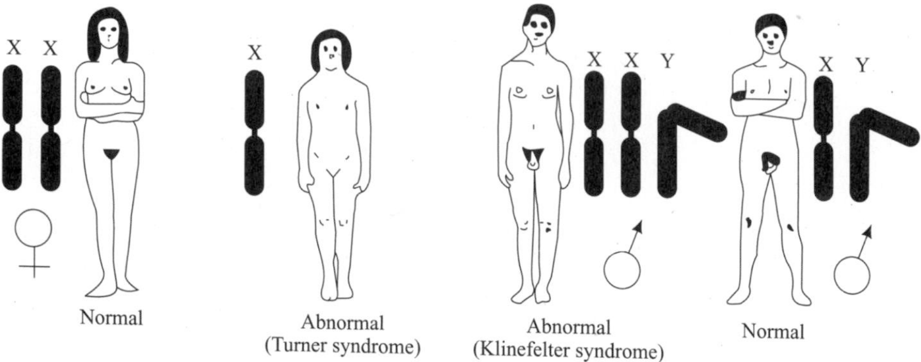


**Fig. 9.15** Turner and klinefelter syndrome
(Source : www.emc.maricopa.edu)

### 4. Euploidy

Euploid organisms have varying number of complete haploid chromosomal sets. Gametes are haploids (n) and somatic cells are diploids (2n). Organisms with higher number of sets, such as triploids (3n) and tetraploids (4n) are called polyploids.

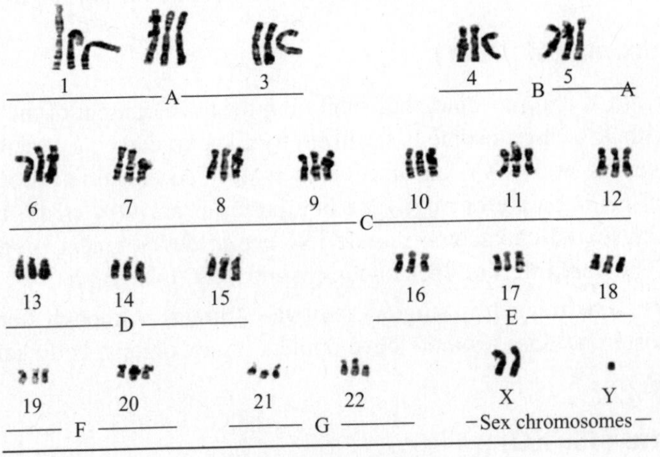

**Fig. 9.16** Triploidy
(Source : www.asklenore.com)

Three kinds of problems arise due to polyploidy. (i) There exists a general imbalance of genetic material being excess. (ii) The chromosomal sex determining mechanism is disrupted. (iii) Meiosis produces imbalanced gametes.

Only a few human polyploids have been reported, and most died within few days of birth. Triploidy is seen in about 10% of all spontaneously aborted human fetuses.

CHAPTER 10

# Genetic Diseases

## INTRODUCTION

Metabolic processes are mediated by enzymes. Enzymes are proteins produced under genetic control and any change in the gene, alter the products of metabolism. **Sir Archibald Garrod,** suggested that most of the hereditary diseases are caused by metabolic blocks, resulting from abnormality of certain specific enzymes and were responsible for many of the 'inborn errors of metabolism'.

## 10.1 PHENYLKETONURIA (PKU)

Biochemical basis of PKU is well understood of human genetic diseases. The following figure shows steps involved in the metabolism of phenylalanine, a common amino acid. Phenylalanine is one of the essential amino acid and the human body cannot form it from any other substances. It must be supplied through food as in the proteins of some common food such as fish, egg and cheese. The ingested proteins are broken down into constituent amino acids. Some of the released phenylalanine is used in the construction of proteins needed in parts of the body. The excess amino acid is converted into another amino acid tyrosine. This depends on the enzyme phenylalanine hydroxylase.

Tyrosine is not an essential amino acid as it could be derived from another amino acid. Tyrosine is used in many ways; one involved in the formation of melanin pigment, one leading to the formation of the hormone thyroxine, and one leading through various steps ending in the complete breakdown to carbon di oxide and water. Specific enzymes control each step. Interruption of the biochemical steps can occur at various points due to gene mutation causing genetic diseases.

PKU is caused by a rare recessive autosomal mutant gene and the genotype being **pp**. Biochemical block is formed due to the absence of enzyme, **'phenylalanine hydroxylase'**. The expression of PKU is pleiotropic as many phenotypic effects are detectable. PKU is characterized by light hair, skin and eye color, mental retardation and microcephaly. Folling, first reported PKU. It affects 1 in 11,000 newborns. PKU was found to account for about 1% mentally retarded patients in institutions. PKU is also linked to other metabolic blocks.

The given illustration depicts 4 inborn errors of metabolism resulting from enzyme blocks at 4 points in the breakdown of phenylalanine a building block of protein. PKU results from a block in the first step of pathway. A block in the next step is due to the homozygous recessive genotype **aa.** This genotype results in a deficiency of enzymes required to change DOPA (3,4 dihydroxy phenylalanine) into a product essential for melanin formation. This results in accumulation of amino acid tyrosine and deficiency of the pigment melanin, causing the pink eyes, white hair and white skin of **albinism**. A block at a different point may bring about a deficiency of the thyroid hormone and cause a form of cretinism, a disorder resulting in retardation of mental and physical development. A block in the conversion of hydroxyphenylpyruvic acid into its product results in a rare disorder, tyrosinosis which requires no treatment.

The hydroxyphenylpyruvic acid is normally changed by another enzyme to another substance, homogentisic acid. This in turn is converted into maleylacetoacetic acid by another enzyme. A homozygous recessive genotype **hh** causes a block at this step which can be deadly in infancy, and leads to **alkaptonuria**, causing severe joint pain, black deposits(alkaptons) in the urine (black urine), palate, ears and eyes. Alkaptonuria is caused by the absence of **homogentisic oxidase** enzyme.

PKU in newborn can be diagnosed by Guthrie test. In this test a small filter paper disk of dried blood from the infant is prepared. It is placed on top of an agar surface inoculated with a bacterial strain that does not reproduce unless phenylalanine is added to the nutrient medium. After incubation, a halo of bacterial growth around a test disk means that excess phenylalanine is present, and is usually diagnostic of PKU.

PKU can be treated by diet therapy, PKU patients are given low phenylalanine diet comprising of apple, banana, cabbage, carrots, tapioca, corn, sugar, butter and multi-vitamin supplements.

## 10.2 G6PD DEFECIENCY

Glucose -6- phosphate dehydrogenase is an important enzyme of the red blood cell and its deficiency is inherited as an X-linked recessive trait. The gene responsible for the G6PD deficiency is located on X-chromosome.

This enzyme is necessary in the metabolism of carbohydrates. Deficiency of enzyme results in sensitivity to sulpha drugs, anti-malarial drugs (primaquine sensitivity), antipyretics, naphthalene, Fava beans etc. and produce hemolytic anemia. **Favism** is a hemolytic condition produced by eating Fava beans and is caused by G6PD deficiency.

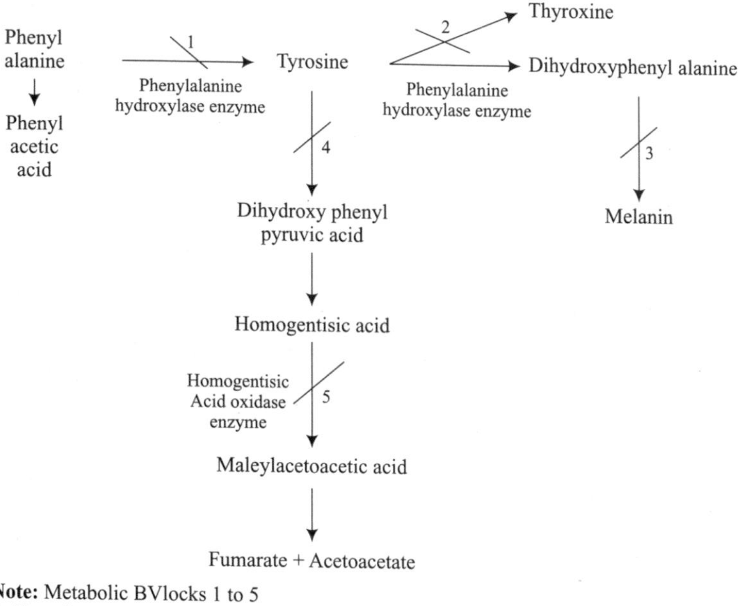


**Fig. 10.1** Metabolic errors in phenylalanine metabolism

It is estimated that more than 150 million people suffer from G6PD deficiency all over the world. In Indian population groups, the association between G6PD deficiency and neonatal jaundice has been well established. The distribution of the deficiency has been shown to be connected with the prevalence of falciparum malaria. It has been suggested that G6PD deficiency confers some resistance to falciparum malaria.

## 10.3 CYSTIC FIBROSIS

It is a lethal autosomal recessive disorder. About 1 in 2500 newborns is affected in Europe. About 1 in 25 is heterozygous and carriers for this disease. There are serious respiratory and digestive problems and extremely salty sweat with high sodium and chloride levels ("salty kisses" in children). Thick, sticky mucus secretion clogs tubules of lungs and other organs causing irreversible damage and malfunctioning of lungs, liver, pancreas, intestine, sweat glands and reproductive organs. Growth is retarded in children. Because of lung problem they are highly susceptible to infection. The gene responsible for this disease is CF and located in long arm of chromosome 7. Average life expectancy for a person with CF is 20 years.

CF can be detected in a child by testing the blood levels of the pancreatic enzyme trypsin which tend to be higher in babies with CF.

The best treatment available includes regular chest physiotherapy to loosen secretions, antibiotics and replacement of digestive enzymes.

## 10.4 DRUG SENSITIVITY

**Pharmacogenetics** is a branch of genetics that deals with the genetically determined variations in drug responses. There is a normal variation in response to all drugs in a population. The specific genes may affect the metabolism of drugs.

Generally when a drug is introduced into the body it passes into the blood stream and gets distributed to various tissues in the body. The drug is either broken down or excreted unchanged by the body. The breaking down process occurs in the liver.

Some enzyme defect can cause extreme sensitivity to certain drugs, which lead to serious clinical problems. If a person having G6PD deficiency take the anti malarial drug **primaquine**, he develops hemolytic anemia. Investigations of unusual inborn drug sensitivities is a rapidly developing area of human genetics called pharmacogenetics.

**Succinylcholine sensitivity** is a genetical based sensitivity. Succinylcholine is used as a relaxant because it interferes with the transmission of nerve impulses and thus decreases muscle activity. In normal people, serum cholinesterase enzyme quickly breaks down the drug. When this enzyme is absent, succinylcholine accumulates at the nerve end for a longer time. Under these conditions, the effects of the drug increase and relaxation turns into a total paralysis.

**Isoniazid** is a drug used in the treatment of tuberculosis. Based on the rate of metabolism of isoniazid, a population can be classified into rapid inactivators, who are homozygous or heterozygous for a dominant allele producing isoniazid inactivating enzyme and slow inactivators who are homozygous for the recessive gene. Slow inactivation of this drug is because of lack of the hepatic enzyme acetyltransferase. This enzyme usually acetylates isoniacid as one step in its metabolism. The slow inactivators may develop neurological problems because of the length of time the drug remains in their system in an active state.

In some persons Coumarin anticoagulants are needed in much higher dosage than normal. This is due to dominant gene which increases the drug ressistance.

Anesthetic agents like halothane and succinylcholine bring about a rare complication of anesthesia namely malignant hyperpyrexia in some individuals. The basic defect in this disorder is a reduced uptake and binding of calcium ions to the sarcoplasmic reticulum. This trait is inherited as an autosomal dominant trait.

## 10.5 DISORDERS ASSOCIATED WITH HAEMOGLOBIN

### a. Sickle Cell Anemia (HbSS)

This is one of the abnormal variant of adult haemoglobin. The red blood cells are sickle shaped. This is caused by a gene mutation which alters the quality of the globin. The haemoglobin has four polypeptide chains in its protein part. In sickle cell anemia one of the amino acids is altered in the beta-globin of the haemoglobin. In the normal haemoglobin the $6^{th}$ amino acid is glutamic acid while in sickle cell it is substituted by valine by changing the codon GAG to GTG. Persons with sickle cell anemia have an abnormally large DNA fragment when the beta globin gene is cut with appropriate restriction enzyme.

This disease resulting from homozygous recessive condition, is a hemolytic anemia (shortened life span of red blood cell) leading to severe anemia. This disease is further characterized by enlarged spleen, painful cries, organ damage, impaired mental functions, increased susceptibility to infection and early death. These blood cells block the vessels and disturb normal circulation in blood vessels.

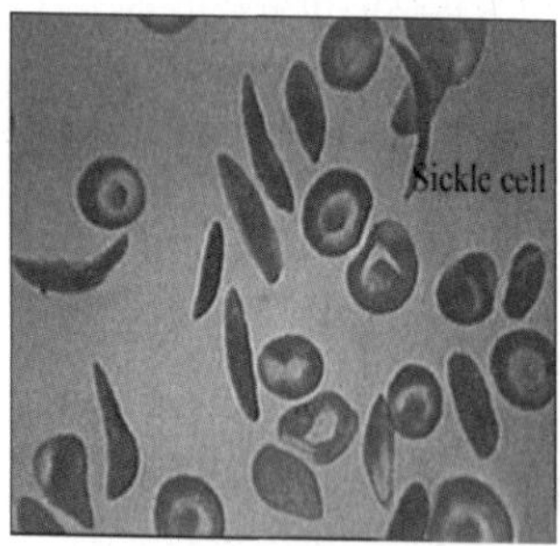


**Fig. 10.2** Normal red blood cells and sickle cells (Source: www.nmh.com)

The wild type is HbAA. The heterozygous condition (HbAS) is termed sickle cell trait. The inheritance of sickle cell disease obeys the principles of Mendelian inheritance. The offsprings of the cross HbAS × HbAa have equal chance of either normal (HbAA) or sickle cell trait (HbAS). If both parents have sickle cell trait (HbAS × HbAS) then the offsprings have 50% chance of sickle cell trait; 25% chance of sickle cell anemia (HbSS) and 25% chance of normal (HbAA).

Very high frequency of sickling has been reported from various parts of south, western and central India. It has been estimated that over 500000 persons among tribals alone are carriers of this genetic disorder and over 200000 are homozygous.

The following steps should be taken for the prevention and treatment of sickling crisis.

The patient should be kept warm, avoid cold and drinking cold water. To avoid dehydration adequate fluid must be taken and excessive heat is avoided. Clot formation within the blood vessels may be prevented by using drugs. Blood transfusion is given when the haemoglobin level falls. Prophylactic antibiotics are given to prevent infection.

## b. Thalassemia

Thalassemias are haemoglobinopathies and represent a group of disorders affecting haemoglobin synthesis. This is a common disorder affecting many people in India where the production of normal haemoglobin is inhibited. The two commonly found thalassemias are **beta thalassemia** in which beta-globin chain synthesis is reduced and **alpha thalassemia** where alpha-chain synthesis is affected. Both can exist in homozygous or heterozygous state.

Beta thalassemia in homozygous state is known as **thalassemia major** or **cooley's anemia**. In this disorder red cells of varying size with distorted forms termed as poikilocytes occur. Severe anemia occurs requiring frequent blood transfusions and is often fatal in early childhood. RBC count is much reduced. Splenomegaly is found.

Beta thalassemia in heterozygous state is known as **thalassemia minor** or **cooley's trait**. These people are perfectly healthy.

Alpha thalassemia is a rare disease. In alpha thalassemia major, both alpha chains production are affected and the condition is **hydrops fetalis** which is total. Alpha thalassemia minor (heterozygous state) is harmless.

Thalassemia in some form or other is one of the most important hemoglobinopathy in India. It has been reported from almost all regions and is clearly most widespread. Several studies have brought to light a large number of subjects with thalassemia in various forms.

The only treatment for thalassemia is regular blood transfusions, usually every four week and bone marrow transplant. Drug Desferal is given to remove excess of iron when blood transfusion is done frequently.

## 10.6 COLOUR BLINDNESS

This term is usually applied to those who cannot perceive colours. Most commonly observed type is red/green colour blindness. This is a standard example of sex-linked recessive inheritance in man and is harmless. The only problem with colour blindness is that the persons afflicted with colour blindness can not be employed in Airways and Railways. Persons who cannot see red belong to **protanopia** type and who cannot see green belong to **deutranopia** type.

The prevalence rate of colour blindness has been found to be highest in western India, followed by Southern, Northern, Central and Eastern India.

The genotypes and phenotypes are given below:

- XA = normal vision
- Xa = colour blind

The possible genotypes and phenotypes of males and females are:

- XA Y = a male with normal vision
- Xa Y = a male with colour blindness.
- XA XA = female with normal vision
- XA Xa = a carrier female with normal colour vision
- Xa Xa = a female who is colour blind (only if mother is carrier and father is colour blind)

Because daughters have two X chromosomes, they are almost always unaffected (heterozygotes). The normal allele "masks" the mutated allele. Colour blind females are rare because they must inherit two recessive alleles for colour blindness.

Males show the trait much more often than females do because they only inherit **one** allele - from their mother and they receive it through X choromosome - if that one is mutated, they will be colour blind.

## 10.7 HAEMOPHILIA

It is a sex linked recessive disorder. In this condition, absence or deficiency of a specific protein clotting factor greatly slows blood clotting. In haemophilia A or Royal haemophilia, clotting factor viii, namely anti haemophilic globulin is absent and in haemophilia B or Christmas disease, clotting factor ix, the christmas factor is absent. A cut may take a long time to stop bleeding. Haemophilia is passed from a carrier (heterozygous) mother to affected son with a risk of 50%. A daughter has a 50% chance of inheriting the mutant allele and is a carrier, like her mother.

The disorder has appeared in the royal families of England, Germany and Russia. The mutant allele apparently arose in Queen Victoria who was a carrier.

Males are **hemizygous** (one allelic for X chromosome) and the incidence being about 1/10,000 male birth. Female homozygotes are very rare and is about 1/100 million. Haemophilia is no longer a mysterious disease in India. 50,000 to 60,000 severe haemophilics were found in India.

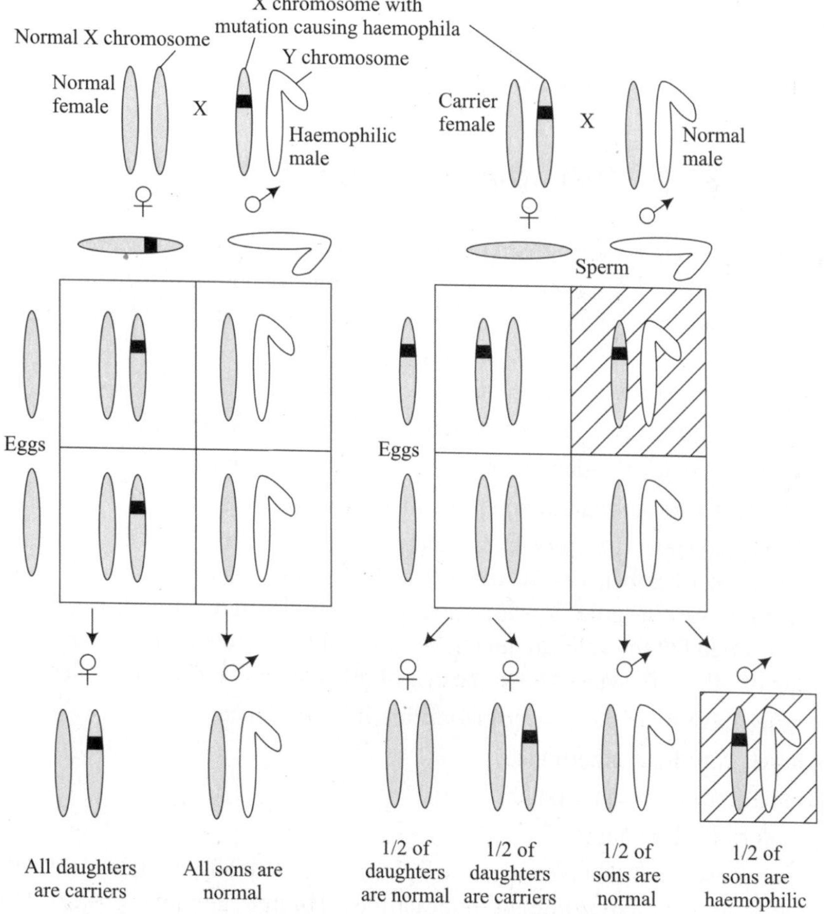


**Fig. 10.3** Inheritance pattern of haemophilia (Source: www. accessexcellence.org)

Regular blood transfusion is usually done to treat haemophilia. A patient requires 25 units of the blood clotting factor per Kg of his body weight. However HIV and hepatitis are risk factors.

Carrier detection and prenatal testing are done to prevent the occurrence. In India the Institute of Immunohaematology at CMC, Vellore is recognized by the World Federation of Haemophilia as an international training center.

## 10.8 DUCHENNE MUSCULAR DYSTROPHY (DMD)

DMD is an X-linked recessive disease occurring in about 1 in 3,500 newborn males. The normal muscle protein **dystrophin** is absent. Usually the onset occurs before age 6 years, and the victim is chair ridden by age 12 and dead by age 20. The earliest signs are delays in walking and talking. Then come weakness and gradual wasting of thigh and pelvic muscles, leading to unsteadiness, difficulty in walking stairs or rising from chairs. As the shoulder, trunk and back muscles gradually weaken and degenerate, the child develops a 'swayback' posture, has trouble maintaining balance and falls a lot. Heart problems are the rule, sometimes leading to sudden death. DMD is often caused by a break in the short arm of X chromosome i.e. xp 21.

## 10.9 DIABETES MELLITUS

This disease is a faulty sugar metabolism due to lack of hormone insulin secreted by beta cells of pancreas. It is characterized by increased sugar level and weakness. Frequent urination is often present. The age of onset may vary from childhood to very old age. The expression of the disease may also vary.

There are two major types of Diabetes:

Type I, is insulin dependent and often called juvenile diabetes

Type II, is non-insulin dependent, and often called adult onset.

There is also gestational diabetes occurring only in pregnancy.

In Type I, the pancreas does not make enough insulin. Without taking insulin the affected person will die, Type II diabetes is 10 times more prevalent than Type I. It is one of the most common chronic diseases in India. It is associated with obesity and aging. It is a life-style disease. Here insulin is secreted but the cells are unable to utilize it for metabolizing sugar. Incidence is high in the age group of 40 to 70 years. Above the age of 50 years it is more in females than in males.

Three theories have been put forward regarding its inheritance:

i. Autosomal dominant inheritance
ii. Autosomal recessive inheritance
iii. Multifactorial inheritance

Studies have shown that diabetes is not simple; it is genetically complex, involving multiple genes, and multiple gene-environment interactions. Human genome project has identified chromosome 2 carrying a gene locus showing susceptibility to Type II diabetes. Two new susceptibility genes have been localized in 11q and 6q.

## 10.10 HYPERTENSION

Hypertension is the measure of pressure or tension exerted by the blood on the walls of arteries and elevated level of pressure is called hypertension or high blood pressure. In a normal adult, blood pressure rises to a peak value (Systolic pressure) 120 mmHg in each cardiac cycle and falls to a minimum value (diastolic pressure) of about 70 mmHg. High blood pressure is 140/90 mmHg. Hypertension affects 25% of the world's adult population and is a major risk factor for stroke, myocardial infarction and heart and kidney failure. Although scientists have believed this condition to be hereditary, it is the result of combination of hereditary and environmental factors. It has been identified in Human genome project that there are genes in chromosomes 2, 5, 6 and 15 responsible for high blood pressure.

## 10.11 HYPERCHOLESTEROLEMIA

Hypercholesterolemia is common disease affecting 1 in 500 worldwide, accounting for 5% of all heart attacks, is showing autosomal dominant inheritance.

Cholesterol is a major component of cell membranes and is the raw material for bile acids and steroid hormones. Cholesterol is needed in our bodies. The body gets cholesterol in two ways; from food and what liver cells can produce. In the intestine fats are broken down into cholesterol and triglycerides. Since they are insoluble in water they are transported as lipoprotein particles. Cholesterol is carried by low density lipoprotein (LDL) fraction. The cell membrane has LDL receptors which pulls the LDL into the cytoplasm. But if cholesterol is in excess the regulatory mechanism is impaired and cholesterol remains in the blood and gets deposited on the artery walls resulting in atherosclerosis and heart disease.

The LDL receptor is a protein made up of 839 amino acids. The LDL receptor gene is present in the short arm of chromosome 19.

## 10.12 BLOOD GROUP INCOMPATIBILITIES AND RELATED DISEASES

In 1900 Karl Landsteiner determined the types of blood and explained the ABO blood group and incompatibilities. The ABO blood type is determined by I genes with three alleles, IA, IB and i. IA IA and IA i individuals are blood type A, and have antigen A in their RBC. $I^B$ $I^B$ or $I^B$ i genotypes are of blood type B with antigen B in their RBC. People with genotype IA IB are of blood type AB and have antigen A and B in their RBC. Those with genotype ii have O blood type and no antigens in their RBC.

Blood type incompatibility occurs when a person's immune system manufactures antibodies that attack the antigens not on his or her cells. A person with blood type A, for example, has antibodies against type B antigen. If he or she is transfused with type B blood, the anti-B antibodies cause the transfused red blood cells to clump and block circulation.

ABO blood type is often followed by a 'positive' or 'negative' which refers to another blood group antigen, the Rh antigen. If one has Rh antigen he or she is Rh positive and if not he or she Rh negative. This is determined by alleles of three genes called C, D and E. The Rh antigen was originally identified in rhesus monkeys, hence the name.

**Table 10.1** ABO blood types

| *Genotype* | *Phenotype* | *Antigen* | *Antibodies* | *Can donate to* | *Can receive* |
|---|---|---|---|---|---|
| $I^A I^A$ or | Type A | A | anti-B | A, AB | O, A |
| $I^A i$ | | | | | |
| $I^B I^B$ or | Type B | B | anti-A | B, AB | O,A |
| $I^B i$ | | | | | |
| $I^B I^B$ | Type AB | A,B | none | AB | all |
| ii | Type O | O | anti-A, anti-B | all | O |

The Rh blood group incompatibilities is the result when a woman who is Rh negative marries a man who is Rh positive, the first born child of such a marriage is usually normal. However, during the following pregnancies the fetus may be lost by still birth or it may be born in such an anemic or jaundiced state that it lives only a few hours or days after birth. The infant dies from **Erythroblastosis fetalis,** a condition of anemia due to the break down of RBC (haemolysis) in the fetus and jaundice. The blood vessels in the liver become clogged with the broken RBCs and the condition is called haemolytic jaundice. This is in response to destruction of baby's RBC by the maternal Rh antibodies. In some cases babies may still born or may die shortly after delivery.

The blood vascular system of mother and child are quite separate. Any exchange of nutrients or other metabolic products between mother and child takes place by diffusion across the placenta. Placenta is an effective barrier which restricts the passage of most substances other than those directly involved in the normal development and growth of the offspring. However at times, capillaries of the placenta may become defective so that they break or allow the seepage of blood from the fetus into that of the mother. If Rh positive blood from fetus enters the circulatory system of Rh negative mother, the response is the formation of antibody against Rh positive blood. The antibodies from the mother may then pass back across the placenta. Generally, the antibodies produced on the first pregnancy are not sufficient to produce serious effect. The second pregnancy will increase the antigen level. In this case the fetus RBCs will be destroyed causing erythroblastosis fetalis.

In this condition a newborn infant may be given blood transfusion to replace the blood with damaged RBCs. Antibodies against Rh antigen namely Rh immunoglobulin (Rhogam) is given to the mother within 36 hours of delivery of child. This will destroy any Rh positive fetal red cells that might have entered maternal circulation and prevents Rh sensitization against later Rh positive pregnancy.

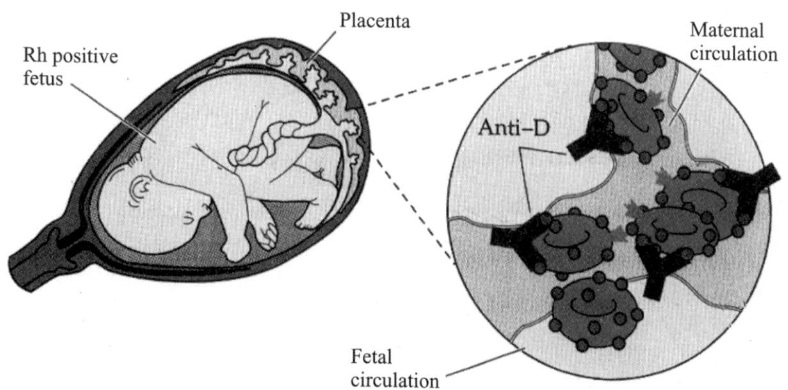


**Fig. 10.4** Protection against erythroblastosis fetalis (Adapted from Mangae E.J. and A.P. Mangae, 1999)

## 10.13 INTERSEXES

Intersex condition is one in which the genitalia are ambiguous and the sex character of the patient may not be according to his or her chromosome pattern. There are two ways of expression of intersex. One is true hermaphroditism and the other is pseudohermaphroditism.

A true hermaphrodite is an individual who has the reproductive organs of both sexes. The external genital differentiation is usually incomplete and anomalous. The gonad may be ovary or testis separately or combined in an ovo-testis. Externally they are more male. 80% of the patients develop gynecomastia and about 50% of the patient mensturate. There is mosaiscism with regard to chromosomes. The individuals have more than one kind of chromosome complement for example 46xx/47xxx; 45xo/46xx; 46xx/48xxyy etc.

Pseudohermaphroditism if seen in male there is 'testicular feminization'. These patients are phenotypically and physiologically y males who are amenorrheic and infertile. There is no sperm production. The chromosome complement is normal. If it occurs in a female the development of internal genital organs are normal while the external genitalia show varying degrees of virilization. There is primary amenorrhea.

## 10.14 CONSANGUINEOUS MARRIAGES AND GENETIC DISEASES

There is a widespread belief that the children of consanguineous marriages (marriages between related individuals) are much more likely to suffer from malformations and genetic diseases. The nature of consanguinity consists of the fact that relatives, because they have common ancestors, possess a greater number of common genes. The number of common genes depends upon the degree of relationship. For example, the share of common genes due to common ancestry in the case of—

i. identical twins (Monozygotic twins) =1;
ii. parent-children=1/2;
iii. uncle-niece/aunt-nephew =1/4;
iv. first cousins=1/8;
v. second cousins=1/32.

The increased risk of homozygosity for deleterious genes and reduction in heterozygosity among the children of related (specially first cousins) is manifested as early fetal death, congenital malformations, mental defects, deaf-mutism, albinism, phenylketonuria, xeroderma pigmentosum, total colour blindness, etc.

CHAPTER 11

# Cancer and Heredity

## INTRODUCTION

Cancer is the second more frequent cause of death after heart disease. Certain people may have a genetic predisposition to cancer. Many environmental factors such as ionizing radiation, exposure to mutagenic chemicals and viruses, nutritional excesses or deficiencies contribute to increased risk of cancer formation.

Cancer can be defined as the unregulated growth and production of cells. Often these cells are incompletely differentiated. Cancers can be subdivided into leukemias and lymphomas, cancer of white blood cells; sarcomas, cancer of bone and muscle cells; and carcinomas, cancer of skin. Benign tumors are non-cancerous growth and remain localized and can be removed surgically. Malignant tumors may spread throughout the body threatening patient's life. This process of migration of cells is called metastasis.

## 11.1 CANCER AS A GENETIC DISEASE

Most of the human cancers are not hereditary and not contagious. Cancer cells have been genetically altered in one or more ways. There are abundant experimental evidences to support the idea that somatic mutations can cause the conversion of a normal cell into a cancer cell. Somatic-cell mutations are not passed on to progeny; so it is not possible that most cancer can be inherited.

The idea that cancer begins with genetic changes is supported by the study on a rare human skin cancer, **Xeroderma pigmentosum**. The skin cells of these persons contain a mutant gene and consequently lack the enzymes involved in DNA repair that has been damaged by UV light. People with this hereditary disease when exposed even to slight amounts of sunlight develop skin tumors.

**Table 11.1** Oncogenes and human cancers

| *Oncogene* | *Cancer* | *Translocation (t) Between Chromosomes** |
|---|---|---|
| myc | Burkitt lymphoma | 8:14 |
| Myc | T cell leukemia | 8:14 |
| bcl-1 | Chronic B-cell leukemia | 11:14 |
| bcl-2 | Follicular lymphoma | 14:18 |
| Abl | Mylogenous leukemia | 9:22 |
| Abl | Lymphocytic leukemia | 9:22 |

*The oncogene is observed to undergo translocation (t) from its original chromosomal location (the first number) to another chromosome (the second number).

Alfred Knudson proposed in 1971, a model to explain the genetic basis of cancer. He explained that in retinoblastoma (eye cancer) two separate genetic defects are required to develop cancer of the eye. In the cases in which the disease affects only one eye, a single cell in one eye undergoes two successive mutations. Because the chance of these two mutations occurring in a single cell is remote, retinoblastoma is rare and typically develops in only one eye. If the cancer is in both the eyes, Knudson proposed that the child inherited one of the mutations and so every cell contains this initial mutation. To develop cancer a second mutation is all that is required. Since each eye possesses millions of cells, there is a high probability that the second mutation will occur in at least one cell of each eye, producing tumors in both eyes at an early age.

The given explanation suggests that cancer is a multistep process that requires several mutations. If one or more of the required mutations is inherited, fewer additional mutations are required to produce cancer, and the cancer will tend to run in families.

It is recognized that cancer is fundamentally a genetic disease, although few cancers are actually inherited. Most tumors arise from somatic mutations that accumulate during life time either through spontaneous mutations or in response to environmental mutagens.

Cancer begins when a single cell undergoes a mutation that causes the cell to divide at an abnormally rapid rate. The cell divides giving rise to a clone of cells, each carrying the same mutation. Because the cells of the clone divide more rapidly than normal, they soon outgrow other cells. Additional mutations that arise in the clone may further enhance the ability of those cells to proliferate, and cells carrying both mutations become dominant in the clone. Eventually, they may be overtaken by cells that contain yet more mutations that enhance proliferation. In this process called **clonal evolution**, the tumor cells accumulate more mutations that allow them to become increasingly more aggressive in their proliferative properties.

Any genetic defect that allows more mutations to arise will accelerate cancer progression. Genes that are involved in DNA repair are often mutated in cancers. Mutations in genes that affect chromosome segregation also may contribute to the clonal evolution of tumors. Many cancer cells are aneuploid and chromosome mutations contribute to cancer progression by duplicating some genes and eliminating others.

## Genes Involved in Cancer

Cell division is regulated by two kinds of signals, one that stimulate cell division and the other that inhibit it. In normal cells these control mechanisms are applied at the same time, and so cell division proceeds in proper speed. The stimulatory genes that cause cancer are termed **oncogenes**. More than 70 oncogenes have been discovered. Cell division may be stimulated when inhibitory genes are made inactive. Inhibitory genes in cancer are termed **tumor-suppressor genes**. Oncogenes or mutated tumor suppressor genes are required to produce cancer. The tumor-suppressor gene to be identified first is the retinoblastoma gene.

Oncogenes were the first cancer causing genes to be identified. The first oncogene, called src, was first isolated from the Rous sarcoma virus in 1970. In 1975 Michael Bishop, Harold Varmus, and other colleagues discovered that genomes of all normal cells carry DNA sequences that are closely related to viral oncogenes. These cellular genes are called **proto-oncogenes**. They are responsible for basic cellular functions in normal cells but, when mutated, they become oncogenes that contribute to the development of cancer. When a virus infects a cell, a proto-oncogene may get incorporated into viral genome through recombination. The proto-oncogene may mutate within the viral genome into an oncogene that, when inserted back into a cell causes rapid cell division and cancer. Proto-oncogenes can be converted into oncogenes in viruses by different ways. The proto-oncogene sequence may be altered when incorporating into viral genome. This mutated copy then produces an abnormal protein that causes cancer. Through recombination, a proto-oncogene may lie near a viral promoter or enhancer, which causes the over expression of the gene. Lastly, sometimes the function of a proto-oncogene is altered when virus inserts its DNA into the gene, disrupting its normal function.

Genes that control the cell cycle often serve as proto-oncogene or tumor-suppressor genes. The cell cycle is regulated by **cyclins** whose concentration varies during cell cycle and cyclin-dependent kinases (CDK) which have a constant level during cell cycle. Genes that encode cyclins and factors that inhibit or stimulate the formation of activated CDKs are often oncogenes and tumor-suppressor genes respectively. Mutated cyclin genes have been associated with cancers of the breast, digestive system and immune system. In many cancer cells genes p16 and p21 that encode CDK are missing.

Cells undergo **apoptosis** when they are damaged or abnormal. Cancer cells often mutate and stimulate apoptosis and prevent their proliferation. Often these cells have mutations in the genes that regulate apoptosis, and they therefore do not undergo programmed cell death. The ability of a cell to undergo apoptosis in response to DNA damage, depends on a gene namely p53, which is inactive in many cancer cells.

Cancer arises by accumulation of multiple mutations in a single cell. The mutation rate often depends upon DNA repair systems. Defects in genes that control DNA repair system is often noticed in a variety of cancers. The examples for this kind of defects are Xeroderma pigmentosum, colorectal, endometrial and stomach cancers.

Most tumors contain cells with a variety of chromosome abnormalities, like an extra chromosome, loss of a chromosome and chromosome rearrangements. In normal cell cycle there are **check points**, responsible for assembly of mitotic spindle. Aneuploid cancer cells contain mutant genes that encode proteins involved in check points. In these cells anaphase proceeds without a proper assembly of mitotic spindle and thereby chromosome abnormalities occur.

In addition to controlling apoptosis, the tumor-suppressor gene p53 plays a role in duplication of centrosome, required for proper formation of spindle and for chromosome separation. Usually the centrosome replicates only once in a cell cycle. If p53 is mutated or missing, the centrosome may undergo extra duplications, resulting in abnormal segregation of chromosomes.

An enzyme called **telomerase** is also involved in cancer formation. Telomeres are sequences that are found at the ends of eukaryotic chromosomes. The ends of the chromosomes are usually not replicated and telomeres become shorter with each division. This shortening leads to chromosome destruction and cell death. S. Somatic cells are capable of limited number of cell divisions. But in germ cells telomerase replicates the chromosome ends and maintains the telomeres. This enzyme is not found in somatic cells. In many tumor cells the gene for telomerase is mutated and so the enzyme is expressed and the cells divide uncontrollably.

There are a set of factors like oxygen and nutrients that are necessary for growth of tumors. The growth of new blood vessels namely angiogenesis is important in tumor progression. This process is stimulated by growth factors and proteins which are encoded by genes whose expression is precisely regulated. In tumor cells these genes are often over expressed and inhibitors of angiogenesis are inactivated or under expressed.

## 11.2 HERITABLE CANCERS

**Retinoblastoma** is a cancer of retina occurring in one or both the eyes. The frequency is about 1 in 20,000 persons. This malignant tumor develops in young children. The symptom is the glassy appearance of the pupil of the eye. It metastasizes and affects other organs causing early death. About 40% of cases run in families and heritable; 60% cases occur sporadically and are non heritable. Heritable cases are caused by a deletion in chromosome 13q where the normal gene Rb is located.

**Wilms tumor** is a cancer that develops in the embryonic cells of one or both the kidneys. The frequency is 1 in 10,000 children. A dominant gene Wt may affect both the kidneys. A deletion in 11q causes this tumor.

**Ataxia-Telangiectasia (AT)** is an autosomal recessive disease and the frequency is 1 in 40,000 children. The gene responsible for AT is pleiotropic. Affected infants show several symptoms. Ataxia refers to loss of muscle control due to progressive damage of the brain. Telangiectasia refers to skin redness due to dilation of capillaries. The patients develop malignancies, especially lymphomas, leukemias and carcinomas of stomach, ovary, breast and other organs.

**Chronic myelogenous leukemia (CML)** affects many people and the chromosomal marker is Philadelphia chromosome, a reciprocal translocation between long arms of chromosomes 9 and 22.

**Burkitt lymphoma (BL)** is occurring mainly in Africa is a malignancy of B lymphocytes. The frequency is 1 in 10,000 children. The solid tumors affect the bones of the jaws and the organs in the abdomen. It is extremely fast growing and aggressive. The BL is due to a translocation involving the c-myc proto-oncogene at band q24 on chromosome 8. The other chromosome is 14 or 22 or 2.

### Breast Cancer Gene (BRCA1)

Frequent cases of breast cancer would be associated with mutations of BRCA1. This gene is located in q21 of $17^{th}$ chromosome. This gene is a large one spanning about 100,000 bases. Its protein product is of 1863 amino acids. Researches have discovered more than 100 different mutations of BRCAI spread out along the gene. The incidence of breast cancer is 1/500 female. Researchers have found out more than 100 different mutations of BRAC1 spread out along the gene. 60% of these mutations are frame shift, 20% are nonsense, 10% are missense mutations and 10% are mutations in splice sites. Another gene BRCA2 on chromosome 13 was discovered in 1992 causing a breast cancer risk in men.

## 11.3 ENVIRONMENTAL FACTORS AND CANCER

Though cancer is basically a hereditary disease, most cancers are not inherited and are influenced by environmental factors. The environmental agents that initiate cancer in somatic cells are called carcinogens. Most of them induce mutations. About 90% carcinogens are mutagenic.

### a. Radiation

Higher incidence of leukemia among the survivors of Hiroshima and Nagasaki atomic-bomb blasts indicates that atomic radiation is a carcinogen - an agent that causes cancer. UV rays damages DNA by the covalent linking of thymine bases to form dimers and a mutation arise there. Ionizing radiation like, x-rays possess energy to knock electrons out of their orbits around atoms and produce mutations in the DNA of cells.

### b. Chemicals

Many chemicals penetrate cells and interact with DNA, thereby increasing the mutation frequency. Over modern life-style is intimately linked to the use of chemicals. Every day almost everybody uses paints, plastics, pharmaceuticals, pesticides etc. We use polyurethane, foam cushions, plastic combs, pens and wear nylon, rayon and polyester clothes. All of us are exposed to varying amounts of thousands of chemicals used in industry and agriculture. Though most of the chemicals that we use are safe, some are proven carcinogens.

Dietary factors are thought to be responsible for cancer deaths. A number of them are animal carcinogens or they are converted to carcinogens by storage or preparation of foods or by metabolic events in the body. Examples are hydrazines in mushrooms, piperines in black pepper, and pyrrolizidines in herbal tea.

Evidence that certain chemicals cause cancer is reported from the occurrence of cancer among industrial workers. It was observed that a high incidence of bladder cancer in rubber workers; lung cancer among asbestos and arsenic industry workers and liver cancer in the workers of PVC industry. Deaths from lung cancer are almost directly proportional to the number of cigarettes smoked.

CHAPTER 12

# Immunogenetics

## INTRODUCTION

Immune systems give protection against microbes. The study of these protective mechanisms is called Immunology and Immunogenetics is the study of genes that are involved in immune mechanisms. The mechanisms of immunity consist of interactions between numerous cells and molecules. The understanding of these mechanisms is important in the prevention and, diagnosis and treatment of the diseases. Immune system is also vital in blood transfusions and organ transplantation. The growth of Molecular biology has given deeper understanding to the study of immune systems.

## 12.1 IMMUNE FUNCTION

Immunity is provided by mobile white blood cells termed lymphocytes and scavenger cells called macrophages. Lymphocytes are made in the bone marrow and migrate to the lymph nodes, spleen, tonsils and thymus gland, and circulate in the blood and tissue fluid. Macrophages are large, irregularly shaped white blood cells that eat up and digest foreign substances.

Antigens are molecules present in the cell surface that elicits immune response in another individual. Antigens are usually a protein or carbohydrate molecule.

Immune reaction is quick, specific and diverse and most of the times many infections are halted before the symptoms arise. Immune system remembers and produces a response when there is similar infection second time.

When a foreign organism enters, the body encounters it with the first line of defense, i.e., innate immune system formed by phagocytes and the complement system. The innate immune system recognizes the general features of the invading microorganisms. After the first line of defense is a more specialized immune response.

The immune response is of two kinds: 1. **humoral immune response** involving antibody or immunoglobulin and 2. **cellular response** involving T cells.

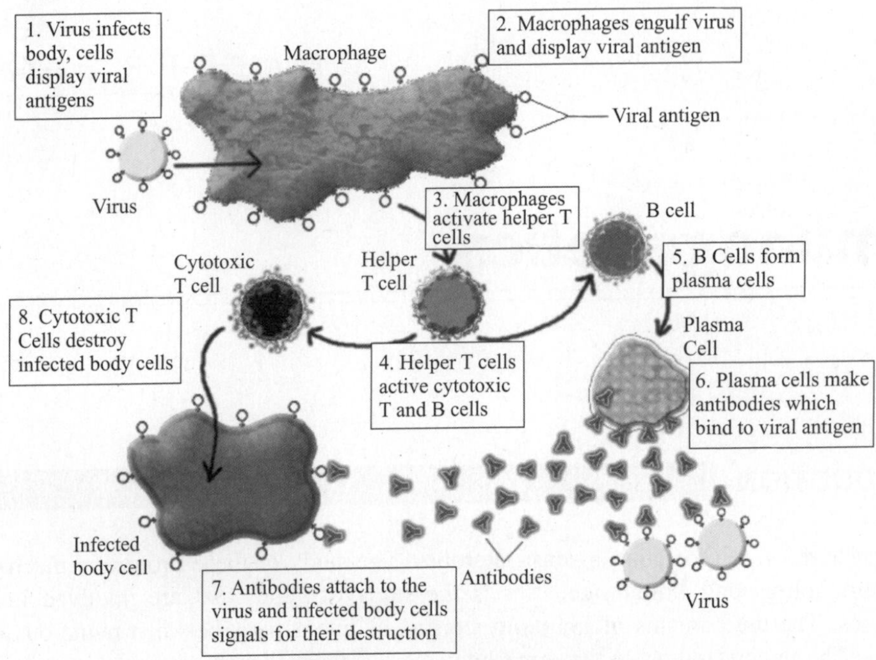


**Fig. 12.1** Immune response
(Source : www.rkm.com.au)

## a. Humoral Immune Response

Humoral response is constituted by the B cells secreting antibodies. B cells which are activated by stimulated T cells divides, and produce clones (group of identical cells) of B cells that can identify the antigen. These cells are either plasma cells or memory cells. A plasma cell exists for few days and secrete continuously about 2000 identical antibodies per second. Plasma cells derived from different B cells secrete different antibodies. The antibodies are specific and correspond to the specific portion of the foreign antigen. The memory B cells respond quickly to the antigen if it invades the body again.

The immune reaction towards the first invasion of the non-self antigen is called primary immune response and it takes a few days. When the infection occurs again there is a faster response called secondary immune response.

## Antibody structure

Antibodies are called **Immunoglobulins (Ig)**. The major form of antibody is **Immunoglobulin G** or gamma globulin. They are large, multipolypeptide proteins, each encoded by several genes. Each molecule is built of four polypeptide chains connected by disulfide bonds to form a shape like the alphabet Y. The two larger polypeptides are called heavy chains (H) and the other two are called light chains (L). Each of the two identical heavy chains consists of four regions of about 110 amino acids each. The regions, called domains, have similar amino acids. Domains similar to heavy chains also occur twice in each of the two identical light chains that are present in the two branches of the Y shaped molecule. The attachment of the branches to the stem of the Y is somewhat flexible. The lower portion of each chain is an amino acid sequence that is identical in all antibody molecules, even in different species. These areas are called constant regions or constant domain (c) . The amino acid sequence of the upper portions of each polypeptide chain, the variable regions or variable domain (v), can differ between antibodies. Most of the variations in amino acids within variable domains is restricted to a few subregions totaling 20 to 30 amino acids. These so called hyper variable regions- three in each light chain and three in each heavy chain form the lining of the antigen-binding cavity. Antibody specificity arises from the three dimensional shape of the cavity and from the particular chemistry of the hypervariable amino acids. The surfaces of the antigen and the heavy and light chains conform like parts of a jigsaw puzzle, but the fit may be either snug or loose.

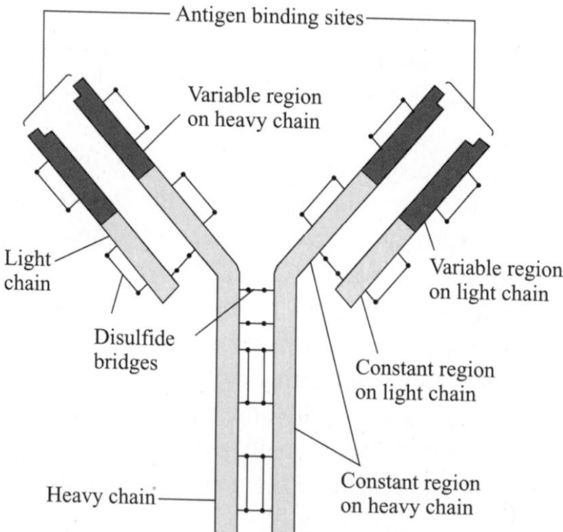


**Fig. 12.2** Structure of antibody
(Source : www.emc.maricopa.edu)

IgG constitutes about 80% of the immunoglobulin molecules. Different immunoglobulin classes G, A, M, E have been analyzed. Each has different amino acids in the stem region of the heavy chains, is found is not only found in plasma but also in body secretions, such as saliva, nasal mucus, sweat and breast milk. IgM has somewhat larger heavy chains than the other classes do, and five of the Y-shaped molecules may be joined together in a circle. IgM molecules bind more firmly to antigens because, each IgM antibody has ten combining sites.

Antibodies can bind to the antigens because of the three dimensional nature of the variable regions. X-ray crystallography images reveal that in antigen-antibody binding, the antibody contorts to form a pocket around the antigen. These specialized ends of the antibody molecule are called antigen binding sites, and the particular parts that actually bind the antigen are called **idiotypes**.

The microbes are inactivated by antigen-antibody binding or the toxin produced by the microorganism is neutralized. Antibodies can cause the pathogens to clump, making them more visible to macrophages, which then destroy them. Antibodies also activate a collection of biochemicals called the **complement system**, which destroys microbes.

## Antibody diversity

The B cells of a person can make a million or more different IgG antibodies each characterized by the distinctive array of amino acids lining the antigen binding pockets. Like any protein, antibodies are encoded by genes. The enormous numbers of antibodies are encoded by a few hundred genes. Several separate DNA sequences are inherited and passed on in germ cells. When they are put together they code for combining sites. To generate diversity, the pieces are shuffled around and combined in different ways during the formation of individual B cells. The shuffling comes out by a process called somatic recombination. Researchers have found that an extended region near the tip of the long arm of human chromosome 14 codes for the heavy chain. There are four families of elements: V (variable), D (diversity), J (joining), and C (constant). During maturation of a particular B cell, intervening DNA regions are cut out, promoting the splicing together, by somatic recombination, of one member each yield unique V-D-J-C gene. The gene is then transcribed and translated into a heavy chain.

The V-D-J portion of the heavy chain gene codes for the variable domain; the C portion codes for all the constant domains, which determine the class of the antibody: IgG, IgM, IgA or IgE. The number of different V-D-J regions that a cell can construct is the product of the number of V, D and J elements. In humans there are approximately 100 V, 20 D and 5 J elements. On the basis of these estimates, $100 \times 20 \times 5 = 10{,}000$ different heavy chain variable domains can be made. The greater number can result from somatic mutation. In this process, base substitution mutations occur at a substantial rate in the immunoglobulin DNA during differentiation of a B cell into a mature plasma cell. To make an antibody, the H chain joins with an L chain from a somewhat similarly processed gene on chromosome 2 to 22 (two different L chain genes). The degree of light chain variation is less, because a V element joins directly with a J element and no family of D element exists.

## Antibody engineering

A single antigen when injected into a mouse generates a mixture of antibodies, each recognizing different part of the antigenic surface. If the antigen is complex, such as a whole virus or cell with a number of proteins, lipoproteins, or glycoproteins on its surface, then hundreds of antibodies will be made, each by a different clone of plasma cells.

Isolating the antibodies is difficult because all the antibodies mix together in the blood plasma. But a special method of making and isolating very homogeneous antibodies with predetermined combining abilities has been demonstrated and it has potential value in the diagnosis and treatment of diseases. Each pure and uniform antibody, called a **monoclonal antibody**, is secreted by a clone of cells grown in culture in unlimited numbers. The special clone is derived by fusing an antibody secreting plasma cell with a cancer cell. The plasma cell becomes immortal because of hybridization. The plasma cell- cancer cell combination is termed **hybridoma.**

Monoclonal antibodies were first developed by German researcher Kohler and Argentina's Cesar Milstein at Cambridge University and were awarded Nobel prizes for this work in 1980.

The basic procedure for generating monoclonal antibodies is outlined in the Figure 12.3.

First, a mouse is injected with the antigen of interest in order to stimulate the proliferation of plasma cells that make antibodies against that antigen. The mouse's spleen, containing a mixture of lymphocytes, is then removed. A suspension of spleen cells, including some activated-antibody producing plasma cells, is mixed with mouse myeloma. The cells grow in medium which allows the growth of fused cells only. Therefore any hybrid cell that is formed will rapidly outgrow the parental cell lines. Several hundred fused cells may be formed from the spleen of one mouse. The resultant clones of cells from each hybrid are isolated and tested for the presence of antibody against the original immunizing antigen. Each isolated hybridoma clone arises from a single plasma cell that secretes a single antibody.

Monoclonal antibodies are used clinically in diagnosing diseases, in cancer therapy, and in blood and tissue typing.

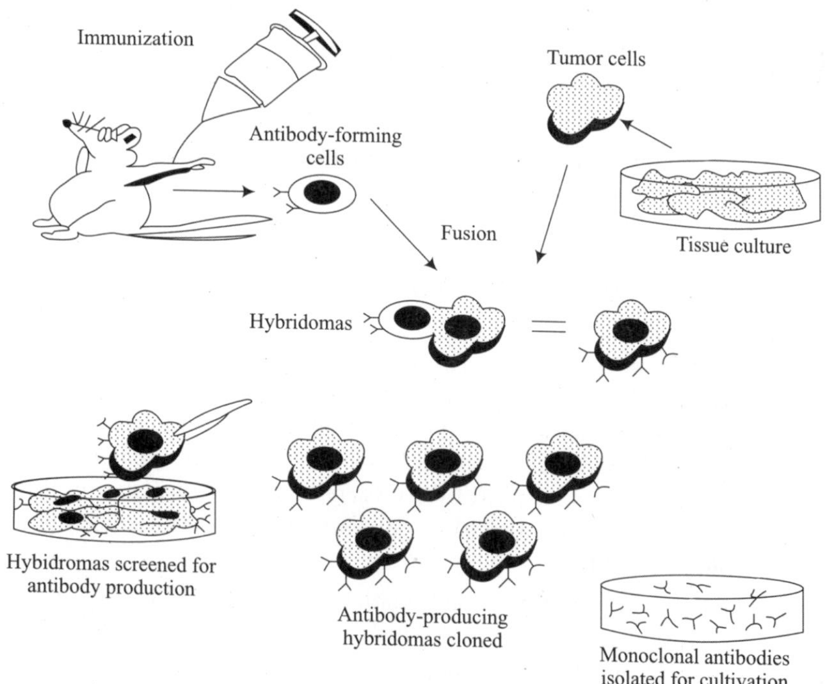


**Fig. 12.3** Monoclonal antibody production
(Source : www.college.ulca.edu)

### b. Cellular Immune Response

**T cells** provide the cellular immune response. Unlike B cells these T cells travel to the sites where they are needed. T cells acquire the ability in the thymus to recognize molecules and cell surfaces. There are several types of T cells performing different functions. Helper T cell stimulates B cells to produce antibodies, secrete **cytokines** and activate another type of T cell called cytotoxic T cell which is also called killer T cell. An immune reaction begins when a helper T cell with a surface protein called a cluster-of-differentiation (CD4) antigen recognizes a macrophage presenting a non-self antigen bound to an HLA glycoprotein. The stimulated CD4 T cell also causes B cells to mature and produce a specific antibody.

The CD4 T cell releases cytokines, including **interleukins, interferons** and **tumor necrosis factor**, which elicit biological response and destroy the invading microorganism. A series of reactions occur when a foreign antigen is encountered by cytokines. For example, interferon binds to a receptor on a cell's surface, which causes 3 proteins in the cytoplasm to join with a fourth in the nucleus. The complete 4-subunit protein is a transcription factor which activates virus-fighting genes.

Cytotoxic T cells attack non-self cells by attaching to them and releasing chemicals. They perform this by using two surface peptides, among many hundreds, which join to form T cell receptors that bind foreign antigens. When a cytotoxic T cell encounters a non-self cell, for example a cancer cell- the T cell receptor draws the two cells together. Then the T cell releases a chemical, **cytolysin**, which drills holes in the foreign cell's membrane. This disrupts the flow of chemicals in and out of the foreign cell, killing it. Cytotoxic T cells are also attracted by their receptors to body cells that are covered with certain viruses, destroying the cells before the viruses spread the infection.

Suppressor T cells inhibit the responses of all lymphocytes to foreign antigens, by closing up the immune response when an infection is controlled.

## 12.2 TISSUE ANTIGENS AND ORGAN TRANSPLANTATION

Organ transplantation is the only alternative left to a patient in the event of non-functioning of vital organs. The main problem with organ transplantation is tissue rejection and the immune system of the body will destroy the foreign tissue if the degree of foreignness is too great. This is avoided by choosing a donor organ with less foreignness. This is done by tissue typing. Such tissue typing identifies the cell surface proteins encoded by a closely linked set of genes on the short arm of chromosome 6, called the human leukocyte antigen (HLA) complex or the major histocompatibility complex or MHC.

The gene products are polypeptides that combine with carbohydrates to form cell surface glycoproteins. Two classes of cell surface molecules are encoded by HLA genes. Class I antigens are encoded by genes B, C, and A; Class II antigens are encoded by several genes within the D region, called DP, DQ and DR. Class I molecules are present on the surface of all nucleated cells in the body, whereas class II molecules are found only on the cells of the immune system.

To be identified by the cells of one's immune system, a foreign antigen may be presented on cell surfaces in conjunction with one's own MHC protein. This recognition step of the immune process is said to be MHC-restricted. This permits immune cells to distinguish 'self' from 'non-self' at once. Helping to discriminate self from non-self is the real function of the protein molecules encoded by the MHC genes.

HLA proteins present foreign antigens on cell surface. Some of the HLA glycoproteins trigger immune response by displaying a non-self antigen on cell's surface. In a process called antigen processing, a viral protein infecting a macrophage is cut into pieces, and transported through the cell's inner membrane network. The viral protein binds to an HLA protein, which then picks up its sugar and travels through the cell membrane to the cell surface.

The macrophage travels with the viral protein to a lymph node, which is the large collection of lymphocytes. When the macrophage's viral and self antigens are recognized by a T cell, other immune reactions are set into motion. The macrophage secretes interleukin-1, which stimulates the T cell to replicate and causes a fever, which may slow viral replication.

HLA genes are the most polymorphic genes known in humans. About 50 different alleles of the B gene, about 10 of the C gene, and about 25 of the A gene control the 85 different antigens.

The HLA genes A, B and C remain in chromosome 6 and are inherited together. The number of possible combinations of these HLA genes is about $50 \times 10 \times 25 = 12{,}500$. A particular combination is called a **haplotype**. The HLA genotype of a person consists of two haplotypes one for each chromosome 6. Considering ABC genes alone there are more than 78 million different HLA genotypes are possible. Since no one genotype is particularly common, no two unrelated people are likely to have exactly the same set of white cell antigens. This great diversity of haplotypes is one reason why organ transplants fail when the donor tissue does not match the receipient.

## 12.3 IMMUNE SYSTEM AND DISEASE

Certain HLA combinations are associated with an increased probability of developing one of 50 or so particular diseases. HLA genes are associated with autoimmune diseases. Example for this is ankylosing spondylitis, an inflammation of the areas where tendons and ligaments attach to bones, especially the bones of the hip and spine. Persons who possessed the HLA antigen B27 increased their risk of the disease 90 times over those who did not have the B27 antigen. In the absence of B27, the disease does not develop.

Many theories have been proposed to explain the correlation between the disease and HLA genes. It may be due to an allele of a gene closely linked to the HLA-B locus. The chromosomes that contain both anklosing spondylitis allele and the HLA-B allele B27 are more common. However, it could be that the polypeptide encoded by the B27 allele simply increases the susceptibility to the disease. Perhaps the B27 antigen is a cell surface receptor for a virus or other pathogen. Alternatively, the B27 molecules may mimic antigens or a pathogen, so that antibodies directed against the pathogen also attack host tissues carrying B27.

Autoimmunity may be obtained by many ways. Sometimes the immune system backfires, manufacturing **autoantibodies** that attack the body's own cells. A virus, perhaps while replicating within a human cell, borrows proteins from the host cell's surface and incorporates them onto its own surface. When the immune system learns the surface of the virus to destroy it, it also learns to attack the human cells that normally bear the particular protein. Another explanation of autoimmunity is that somehow T cells fail to distinguish self from non-self.

A third possible route of autoimmunity is when a non-self antigen coincidently resembles a self antigen. Juvenile Diabetes is example for this. This is a deficiency of the pancreatic hormone insulin, which normally transports glucose in the blood to the cells. Part of protein on insulin producing cells matches part of bovine serum albumin (BSA), which is a protein in cow's milk. Children who are allergic to cow's milk develop antibodies against BSA, which later on attack the similar appearing pancreas cells causing Juvenile Diabetes.

### Immune overreactions

Overstimulation of immune system occurs in a variety of ways. For example the toxins produced by ***Staphylococcus*** act as superantigens. Unusually these superantigens directly combine with MHC molecules and with large number of T cells. The increased number of stimulated T cells responds with an increased amount of **interleukin 2**, which makes people feel ill with nausea, diarrhea and fever.

The by-products of antigen-antibody reactions cause discomforts with allergies. In some people the antigens, or allergens cause immunological reactions when inhaled or eaten or touched or injected even in very small amounts.

Exposure to allergen provokes allergic reactions by B cell leading to circulating antibodies of a special class, IgE. The fast antigen-antibody reaction stimulates certain tissue cells to release histamine. The physiological effects of histamine include contraction of lung muscles and dilation of capillaries. Anaphylaxis, a severe and rapidly developing form of allergy can sometimes be fatal if not quickly treated with histamines.

### Immune deficiencies

The poor functioning of immune system result in certain diseases. These immune deficiency disorders may involve either T cells or B cells or both.

**Agammaglobulinemia** is a rare X-linked recessive disease. Affected child lacks plasma cells and immunoglobulin. Infants suffer from repeated infections. Survival depends on periodic injections of gamma globulin. They possess normal T cells, and patients are no more susceptible to common viral diseases than other infants.

**Severe combined immunodeficiency disease** (SCID) involves the absence of both T cells and B cells. Infants fail to survive because of viral, bacterial and fungal infections and they usually die in the first year. A few SCID patients have been treated with bone marrow transplant. One kind of SCID is **adenosine deaminase deficiency** (ADA deficiency) which is an inherited autosomal recessive disease.

Acquired immune deficiency syndrome (AIDS) is due to the human **immuneodeficiency virus** (HIV), which attacks T cells. Two variants of the virus HIV-1 and HIV-2 are recognized. Immune functions of T cells and B cells gradually deteriorate. Generally no symptoms occur for several months to a year after infection. Usually swollen lymph nodes are the first symptoms. B cells become over active in making antibodies and helper T cells begin to die. Although some of the disease symptoms can be prevented or reduced with medical care and most patients die five to ten years after being infected with HIV.

HIV is a retrovirus containing RNA as the genetic material. On infection it inserts its genome into the viral genome. Large number of new viruses is produced causing the death of the cell. AIDS is transmitted almost entirely by sexual contact or blood exchange and from mother to fetus or nursing baby. Because the virus is highly mutable, treatment is very difficult.

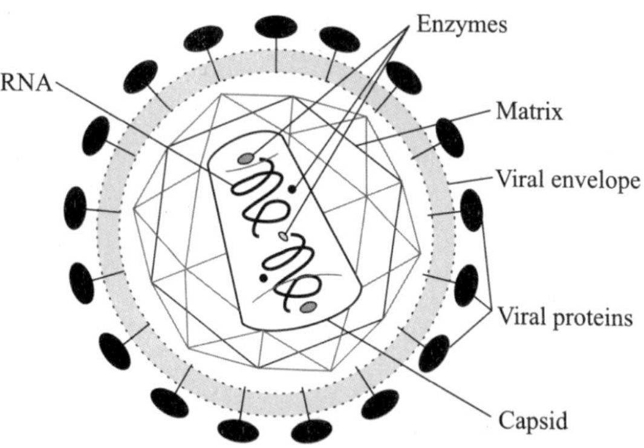


**Fig. 12.4** Structure of HIV
(Source : www.chm.bris.ac.uk)

## 12.4 IMMUNOTHERAPY

Paul Ehrlich developed the concept of magic bullet-a substance that could enter the body and destroy diseased cells. The bio-chemicals and the cells of the immune system are used as magic bullets. The use of immune system to fight against disease is termed immunotherapy.

Monoclonal antibodies (MAb) are used in immunotherapy. MAb can highlight cancer before it can be detected by other means. The MAb is attached to a radioactive chemical, which is then detected when the MAb binds an antigen unique to the cancer cell surfaces.

In cancer treatment drugs or radioactive chemicals are attached to MAbs that are attracted to antigens on cancer cells. When it is engulfed by the cancer cells, they are destroyed.

MAbs are also used to clean bone marrow, the source of many blood-related cancers. Some bone marrow is removed and infused with millions of magnetic beads, each coated with MAbs specific to the cancer cells. When the marrow is passed through a magnet, the cancer cells are pulled out. The clean marrow is then returned to the patient.

### Cytokines

Cytokines are the biochemicals produced by B cells when stimulated by T cells. Interferon was the first cytokine to be tested on a large scale. It is effective against a few types of cancers and multiple sclerosis.

In another approach certain T cells are removed from tumor samples, and incubated with Interleukin-2, which the patient also receives intravenously. The removed T cells, activated by the cytokine, are injected into the patient. This is called lymphokine activated killer, or LAK, cell therapy.

CHAPTER 13

# Population Genetics

## INTRODUCTION

The inheritance of individual genes is governed by Mendelian principles, but the frequencies of these genes in a population may be influenced by many factors like the size of population and frequency of a particular gene and several other factors. The distribution of a particular gene (its alleles) in time and space is not dependent on individuals carrying this gene but is governed by the properties of the population consisting of individuals carrying this gene i.e. its alleles.

A population consists of a community of sexually interbreeding organisms inhabiting geographical region. This population carries particular genes. These populations were called 'Mendelian populations' by Sewall wright, because individuals belonging to these populations follow Mendelian principles of inheritance.

## 13.1 BEHAVIOUR OF GENE IN POPULATION

### Gene Pool and Gene Frequencies

Gene pool and gene frequencies are two important attributes of a population. A **gene pool** is the sum total of genes in gametes of a population. The gene pool is transferred from one generation to the other through the sample drawn from a gametic pool. Gene pool consists of a large number of genes which will vary in their frequencies. **Gene frequencies** are defined as proportions of different alleles of a gene in a population, and in a particular generation these frequencies will depend upon their frequencies in preceding generation. These frequencies also depend on proportion of various genotypes in total population.

For example, in human MN blood groups, in a sample population of 100 individuals with 50 MM, 20 MN and 30 NN, frequencies of 'M' and 'N' can be calculated. Since each individual will have two homologous chromosomes each carrying a particular allele, the frequency of 'M' can be calculated by doubling the number of homozygous 'M' blood group type and adding to it the frequency of heterozygous 'MN' blood group type. In this manner the frequency of 'M' will be $(50 \times 2) + 20 = 120$. Similarly the frequency of 'N' will be $(30 \times 2) + 20 = 80$. The relative frequencies of 'M' allele can be worked as M / M + N and that of 'N' can be worked out as N/M + N. Therefore the frequency of 'M' is 120/200 = 0.6 and that of 'N' is 80/200 = 0.4.

The frequencies of genes can also be worked out with the help of the following formula:

Frequency of gene = frequency of homozygote for that gene + 1/2 frequency of heterozygotes

So frequency of M = 0.5 MM + 1/2 (0.2 MN) = 0.6

frequency of N = 0.3 NM + 1/2 (0.2 MN) = 0.4

## 13.2 HARDY WEINBERG EQUILIBRIUM

In 1908, G.H. Hardy, an English mathematician and W. Weinberg, a German physician independently discovered that an equilibrium is established between frequencies of alleles in a random mating population. It was also shown that the relative gene frequencies remained unaltered from one generation to the next, regardless of their dominance and recessive relationship. This equilibrium was explained by Hardy Weinberg law.

### Frequencies of Two Alleles of a Single Locus

When two individuals heterozygous for the same gene Aa are crossed (Aa × Aa) they segregate in a ratio 1 AA : 2Aa : 1aa. This ratio can be obtained by simple expansion of binomial theorem $(A + a)^2$ = 1 AA : 2Aa : 1aa. In this case, frequencies of A and a are the same i.e. 0.5. The frequencies of 'A' and 'a' are designated as 'p' and 'q'. The probabilities of individuals obtained from random mating from such population can be obtained as shown in Table.

**Table 13.1** Frequencies of three genotypes in a population having allele A and a with frequency p and q respectively

| *Eggs*<br>***Sperms*** | ***A (p)*** | ***a (q)*** |
|---|---|---|
| **A (p)** | AA ($p^2$) | Aa (pq) |
| **A (q)** | Aa (pq) | aa ($q^2$) |

It can be seen in the figure that the probability of homozygous dominant (AA) obtained through random mating would be $p^2$, that of heterozygous (Aa) individuals would be '2pq' and that of homozygous recessive (aa) would be $q^2$. This leads to the formulation of Hardy Weinberg Equation: $p^2$ (AA) + 2 pq (Aa) + $q^2$ (aa). This equation would be obtained in every case after one generation of random mating, if factors like mutation, selection and migration do not separate. In a particular heterogenous population where for a particular character complete dominance is expressed, no distinction between can be made between homozygous dominant (AA) and heterozygous (Aa) individuals. Therefore, 'p' can not be directly determined instead indirectly by 1 – q, by first determining the value of 'q', so that the value of 'q' can be obtained through simple square root of frequency of the individuals having recessive phenotype. Since p + q = 1, p will be equal to 1 – q. Substituting the value 1 – q for p in the Hardy Weinberg equation, it can be written as $(1 - q)^2 + 2q(1 - q) + 1q^2 = 1$.

It is possible to prove algebraically that a population having genotypic frequencies expressed is $p^2 + 2pq + q^2$ will be in equilibrium.

## Assumptions of Hardy Weinberg Equilibrium

1. Population size is effectively infinite,
2. Mating is random in the population (the most common deviation results from inbreeding),
3. Males and females have similar allele frequencies, and the locus is autosomal,
4. There are no mutations and migrations affecting the allele frequencies in the population,
5. The genotypes have equal fitness, i.e., there is no selection (in viability and fitness).

The Hardy-Weinberg law suggests that as long as the assumptions are valid, allele and genotype frequencies will not change in a population in successive generations. Thus, any deviations from Hardy Weinberg law may indicate the following biological processes:

1. Small population size results in random sampling errors and unpredictable genotype frequencies (a real population's size is always finite and the frequency of an allele may fluctuate from generation to generation due to chance events),
2. Assortative mating which may be positive (increases homozygosity; self-fertilization is an extreme example) or negative (increases heterozygosity), or inbreeding which increases homozygosity in the whole genome without changing the allele frequencies.
3. A very high mutation rate in the population (typical mutation rates are $< 10^{-5}$ per generation) or massive migration from a genotypically different population interfere with the allele frequencies.
4. Selection of one or a combination of genotypes (selection may be negative or positive). Selective elimination of homozygotes as in some autosomal dominant diseases, where homozygotes for the mutation may die in utero, is an example (in a very large sample, this could violate HWE). Similar to this selection, sampling error (selection bias) may also affect HWE if bias concerned ethnicity.
5. Unequal transmission ratio (transmission ratio distortion or segregation distortion) of alternative alleles from parents to offspring.
6. Differential gene frequency among males and females.

### Implications of Hardy Weinberg Law

1. The allele frequencies remain constant from generation to generation. This means that hereditary mechanism itself does not change allele frequencies. It is possible for one or more assumptions of the equilibrium to be violated and still not produce deviations from the expected frequencies that are large enough to be detected by the goodness of fit test.
2. When an allele is rare, there are many more heterozygotes than homozygotes for it. Thus, rare alleles will be impossible to eliminate even if there is selection against homozygosity for them.
3. For populations in Hardy Weinberg equilibriuim, the proportion of heterozygotes is maximal when allele frequencies are equal (p = q = 0.50), and when this happens the heterozygote frequency will be 0.50 (2 × 0.50 × 0.50). Unless Hardy Weinberg equilibrium is violated (as in selective loss of homozygotes), heterozygosity can never be more than 0.50 at any biallelic locus.

An application of Hardy Weinberg equilibrium is that when the frequency of an autosomal recessive disease (e.g., sickle cell disease) is known in a population and unless there is reason to believe Hardy Weinberg equilibrium does not hold in that population, the gene frequency of the disease gene can be calculated. Likewise, the carrier rate may be calculated for autosomal recessive disorders if the disease gene frequency is known. For example, phenylketonuria (PKU) occurs in 1/11,000 ($q^2$), which gives a heterozygote carrier frequency of approximately 1/50 [2 × q(1-q) ]. If the diseased individuals ($q^2$) are deducted from the whole population, the carrier rate in normal individuals approximates to [ 2q/1+q ].

## 13.3 CALCULATION OF GENE FREQUENCIES

Distribution of alleles in succeeding generations resulting due to random mating, can be calculated by using Hardy Weinberg equation, $p^2 + 2pq + q^2$. PTC tasting can be taken as an example. The chemical phenylthiocarbamide (PTC) is tasted bitter by some persons. This trait of tasting ability and who can not taste PTC is due to a single gene with two alleles, T and t. Taste trait is controlled by the dominant gene T and the non-taster trait by 't', the recessive gene. Since T is dominant over 't' the tasters can have two genotypes TT and Tt, whereas non-tasters will have only one genotypes 'tt'.

Suppose in an initial population of human beings, different genotypes are represented by ratio 0.40TT : 0.40Tt : 0.20tt. The gene frequencies will be T = 0.40 (TT) + 1/2 × 0.40 (Tt) = 0.60 ; t = 0.20 (tt) + 1/2 × 0.40 Tt = 0.40. The frequencies of T = 0.60 and t = 0.40 will give a genotypic ratio of 0.36 (TT) : 0.48 (2Tt) : 16 (tt) in the next generation. This is illustrated in the Table 13.2.

This has been explained in detail in Table 13.3, where frequencies of different mating types and frequencies of different genotypes in the progeny from each mating type are given. This ratio is obtained when there is random mating. It is visible in the table that although the genotype frequencies have changed, the gene frequencies did not change. This demonstrates that after one generation of random mating, equilibrium in the genotypic ratio can be achieved and this will follow the Hardy – Weinberg equation.

**Table 13.2** Frequency of genotypes of Taster (T) and non-taster (t) under conditions of random mating

| | *p(T) 0.6* | *q(t) 0.4* |
|---|---|---|
| p(T)<br>0.6 | $p^2$<br>0.36 (TT) | pq<br>0.24 (Tt) |
| q(t)<br>0.4 | pq<br>0.24 (Tt) | $q^2$<br>0.16 (tt) |

**Table 13.3** Relative frequencies of the different kinds of offsprings produced by the matings in a population with 0.40 TT, 0.40 Tt and 0.20 tt genotypes

| *Parents* | | *Offspring ratio* | | | *Offspring frequencies* | | |
|---|---|---|---|---|---|---|---|
| *Type of mating* | *Frequency of mating* | *TT* | *Tt* | *tt* | *TT* | *Tt* | *Tt* |
| TT x TT | 0.16 | all 0.16 | | | 0.16 | | |
| TT x Tt | 0.32 | ½ (0.16) + ½ (0.16) | | | 0.16 | 0.16 | |
| TT x tt | 0.16 | all (0.16) | | | | 0.16 | |
| Tt x Tt | 0.16 | ¼ (0.04) + ½ (0.08) + ¼ (0.04) | | | 0.04 | 0.08 | 0.04 |
| Tt x tt | 0.16 | ½ (0.08) + ½ (0.08) | | | | 0.08 | 0.08 |
| tt x tt | 0.04 | all (0.04) | | | | | 0.04 |
| | | Total | | | 0.36 | 0.48 | 0.16 |

### Frequencies of more than Two Alleles at a Single Locus

In the above examples, only two alleles at a single locus is considered. The situation becomes complicated when genes with three or more alleles are taken into consideration.

Each allelic frequency should be considered as an element of multinomial expansion. For instance if there are three alleles, $A_1$, $A_2$ and $A_3$ at the locus, with their corresponding gene frequencies p, q and r, respectively, then $p + q + r = 1$. In such a case the trinomial expansion i.e. $(p + q + r)^2 = p^2 A_1A_1 + 2pq\,A_1A_2 + 2pr\,A_1A_3 + q^2 A_2A_2 + 2qr\,A_2A_3 + r^2$ will represent the genotypic frequencies at the equilibrium stage. This is shown in the Table 13.4.

## 13.4 CHANGES IN GENE FREQUENCIES

Gene frequencies are conserved from one generation to the other under certain conditions. Under these conditions frequencies of genotypes reach an equilibrium after a single generation of random mating. The conditions include absence of **mutation**, **selection**, **migration** and **random drift**. This ideal condition never exists and in a large random (**panmictic**) mating population, changes in gene frequencies do occur. This change can be either directional as in the case of mutation, selection or

**Table 13.4** Frequencies of genotypes when three alleles $A_1$, $A_2$ and $A_3$ are involved with their frequencies being p = 0.2, q = 0.5 and r = 0.3

| | *p(A₁)* *0.2* | *q(A₂)* *0.5* | *r(A₃)* *0.3* |
|---|---|---|---|
| $p(A_1)$ 0.2 | $p^2 = 0.04$ $(A_1A_1)$ | $pq = 0.10$ $(A_1A_2)$ | $pr = 0.6$ $(A_1A_3)$ |
| $q(A_2)$ 0.5 | $pq = 0.1$ $(A_1A_2)$ | $q^2 = 0.25$ $(A_2A_2)$ | $qr = 0.15$ $(A_2A_3)$ |
| $r(A_3)$ 0.3 | $pr = 0.06$ $(A_1A_3)$ | $qr = 0.15$ $(A_2A_3)$ | $r^2 = 0.09$ $(A_3A_3)$ |

migration or non-directional as in the cases of random drifts. The directional change means a change of gene frequencies progressively from one value to another in either direction. If this change proceeds unchecked then fixation of one allele and elimination of the other allele happens. The non-directional change cannot predict the fate of an allele from one generation to the other.

## a. Mutation

Mutation introduces new genes leading genetic differences in the population. These new genes introduced may or may not persist in the population upon their utility. The gene frequencies will also depend upon this factor. This can be illustrated by the following hypothetical example. If a dominant gene 'A' mutates to 'a', then frequency of 'a' will replace 'A'. Quantitatively, let $p_o$ be the initial frequency of 'A' and 'u' be the mutation rate with which 'A' changes to 'a'. In such a case, 'a' will appear with a frequency of $u \times p_o$ in the first generation. The frequency of 'A' will, therefore be reduced by a factor $p_o u$ and become $p_o - p_o u = p_o (1 - u)$. In the next generation there will, therefore, be further change due to the change of A to a, thus further reducing the frequency of A by a factor $p_o (1 - u) - p_o (1 - u) \times u = p_o (1 - u) (1 - u) = p_o (1 - u)^2$. In this manner, in 'n' generations, the frequency of A will be reduced to $p_o (1 - u)^n$. Eventually the term $(1 - u)^n$ will approach zero so that A will disappear after several generations, if no reverse mutation takes place and the mutant allele experiences no selection pressure against it.

However, if the reverse mutation also takes place with a frequency of 'v' and the initial frequency of A and a are $p_o$ and $q_o$ respectively, in one generation the frequency of 'A' will become $p_o + vq_o - up_o$ and that of a will become $q_o + up_o - vq_o$. It is obvious that a gains a fraction $up_o$ and losses a fraction $vq_o$ at the same time. Similarly, a gains a fraction $vq_o$ and loses a fraction $up_o$. Let us now consider the fate of the frequency of 'a' in the following generations. Let the change in the frequency of 'a' be represented as $Dq = up_o - vq_o$. If $p_o$ is relatively larger than $q_o$, and u is relatively larger than V, Dq would be fairly high and the frequency of 'a' i.e., 'q' could increase rapidly. This will lead to a situation, where q becomes larger than p, so that the value of vq will increase and that of up will decrease. As a consequence, q would diminish gradually and at a certain point **'mutational equilibrium'** will be reached where 'Dq' would become zero.

## b. Selection

The gene frequencies may change due to selection in favour of one of the two alleles of a gene. For instance, if individuals with allele A are more successful in reproduction than the individuals with a, the frequency of the former will be higher. The selection can be artificial or natural. The factors influencing selection may include temperature, humidity, food, sexual attractions, etc.

When one genotype can produce more offspring than the other in the same environment, it means relative reproductive success, called **fitness** or **adaptive value** or **selective value**. For instance, if a genotype carrying 'A' produces 100 individuals reaching maturity and another genotype carrying produces 90 individuals in the same environment, this would mean that the reproductive success of 'a' is reduced by 10 % or by a fraction of 0.1. This adaptive value, which is also designated as 'w', ranges from 1.0 for most reproductive genotype to zero for lethals. This may also be expressed in the form of selection coefficient or 'S' which is defined as a force acting on a genotype to reduce its adaptive value. If the adaptive value w is 1, **selection coefficient** 'S' would be zero or **vice versa**. Algebraically, this can be expressed as $w = 1 - S$ or $S = 1 - w$.

## c. Migration

Through migration, new alleles can be introduced into a population from nearby population. Let us consider a large continental population donating individuals (genes) to a small island population. The rate of migration is 'm', which is equal to the fraction of genes on the island that are replaced by genes from the continent each generation. If qi is the frequency of a particular allele 'a', on the island, and qc is the corresponding frequency on the continent, then after migration, the frequency on the island will be $qi = (1 - m)\, qi + mqc$. The change in the frequency of 'a' in one generation will therefore be $\Delta qi = qi' - qi = m\,(qc - qi)$; $\Delta qi$ will become zero either when migration stops ($m = 0$) or when the frequency of 'a' on the island equals the frequency of 'a' on the continent ($qi = qc$).

The effect of migration is to make populations genetically similar. Even a few migrants per generation are sufficient to eliminate the differences among geographically separated populations. Thus, migration can be a powerful homogenizing force.

## d. Random Genetic Drift

This was explained by Sewall Wright and called Sewall Wright effect. The sample of a population, although representative of the population, may not have exactly the same frequency as found in the population. Such deviations in gene frequencies will be due to sampling errors. This again depends on the size of the sample. For instance, if only a few parents are chosen to begin a new population, the gene frequency of this new population may deviate widely from the gene frequencies of the original population, because in this case sampling error will be high. On the other hand, if a large number of parents are taken to begin a new population, deviation in the gene frequencies may not be so large. The deviation in the gene frequency can be measured with the help of standard deviation $\sigma = \sqrt{pq/N}$, where p and q are the original frequencies of the alleles and N is the number of genes sampled. The number of genes sampled will be equal to double the number of individuals due to diploid condition. Therefore the above formula will take the form $\sigma = \sqrt{pq/2N}$, where N is the number of actual parents.

This is illustrated in the following example when p = q = 0.5 and the individuals are 1000. Then σ will be √(0.5 × 0.5)/2000 = √0.25/2000 = 0.011. Therefore the gene frequency of the new population will fluctuate around 0.5 ± 0.011, on the other hand if a new population is started by 2 individuals then σ = √(0.5 × 0.5)/4 = √0.0625, which means the gene frequency will fluctuate around 0.5 ± 0.25 i.e. –0.25 to 0.75. In actual practice, the gene frequencies due to random drift may approach the limit that is zero and one. This would be possible only when new population arises due to a very small sample leading to the fixation of one allele and elimination of the other allele.

$$p + q = 1$$

The Hardy-Weinberg laws rarely holds true in nature (otherwise evolution would not occur). Organisms are subject to mutations, selective forces and they move about, or the allele frequencies may be different in males and females. The gene frequencies are constantly changing in a population, but the effects of these processes can be assessed by using the Hardy-Weinberg law as the starting point.

All discussions presented so far concerns a simple biallelic locus. In real life, however, there are many loci which are multiallelic, and interacting with each other as well as with the environmental factors. The Hardy-Weinberg principle is equally applicable to multiallelic loci but the mathematics is slightly more complicated. For multigenic and multifactorial traits, which are mathematically continuous as opposed to discrete, more complex techniques of quantitative genetics are required.

CHAPTER 14

# Genetics of Behavior

## INTRODUCTION

The genetics of human behavior is an interesting aspect of human biology. Behavior is what people do and how they do it. The actions are expressed by mental or muscular responses to environmental stimuli to the sense organs. The various stimuli are coordinated and controlled by a complicated network of hormonal messengers and nerve impulses. The activities are often affected by proteins. Many proteins are involved in the structure and functioning of the nervous system. When any one of them is altered, there are some alterations in the behavior too. The proteins are encoded by genes. Thus genes, through their products, have the capacity to influence the human behavior. Therefore it is possible that genetic variation can result in behavior variation.

There are many examples to show that single gene mutations influence behavior. The Huntington's disease, an autosomal dominant trait, causes a slow disintegration of the functioning of the nervous system, resulting in a variety of bizarre behaviors. Lesch Nyhan syndrome, a sex linked recessive disorder, is characterized by hyperexcitability of the nervous system leading to self mutilation. Phenylketonuria, an autosomal recessive trait, is characterized by severe mental dysfunction. There are hundreds of single gene loci that in one way or other influence human behavior. Genes influence behavior. But genes do not act in isolation; the environment can modify the genotype.

The genetics of human behavior suffers from lack of experimental evidences. More than a century after Galton raised the question of nature versus nurture, controversies still exist over the contributions of genes and environment. The study of behavior is difficult because there is prolonged interaction of genotype and environment.

## 14.1 ABNORMAL BEHAVIORAL TRAITS

### i. Lesch Nyhan Syndrome

There are several inherited traits that have a behavioral component. One of the well known examples is **Lesch Nyhan syndrome**, characterized by self mutilation is caused by a X linked recessive gene. The normal allele controls the production of an enzyme needed in the metabolism of nucleic acid components. The basic error in this syndrome is a block in purine metabolism. To keep the body cells actively dividing and functioning, the body needs a constant supply of the nitrogenous base making up the genetic code. The purine bases namely adenine and guanine are synthesized by the body from simpler compounds, but it can also be produced by recycling the nucleic acids through salvage pathway. This process is mediated by the enzyme HGPRT. This enzyme is absent in Lesh Nyhan patients. In these patients the nitrogenous bases are not reused but wasted and converted to uric acid. When uric acid accumulates abnormally in the blood and urine, it causes unusual behavior.

Lesch Nyhan babies appear normal. Most of the babies excrete uric acid in their urine, that appears as a red brown or orange 'sand'. At about 6-8 months of age the babies do not show normal physical progress. There may be regression of motor skills. The muscles grow abnormally tight, and the baby exhibits uncontrolled writhing motions and spasms of the trunk and limbs. The legs make 'scissor' walking. Many patients suffer periodic seizures.

The abnormal behavior can be noticed at about two or three years of age. There is compulsive biting and tearing of victim's own lips, mouth, fingers and toes. These children show aggressive behavior towards others also. Their IQ ranges from 30 – 65 classifying them as severely retarded. Most patients exhibit chronic thirst and drink plenty of water. Most of them die during their teen years due to kidney failure or kidney stones.

### ii. Others

Another example of a single-gene behavioral phenotype is **porphyria**, which affected King George III of England. This is a rare autosomal disorder resulting in the defective synthesis of heme, the iron component of the hemoglobin molecule. The symptoms are abdominal pain, constipation, vomiting and wine-red urine. The king suffered from neurological symptoms like visual disturbances and restlessness. Later he became delirious and diagnosed as insanity. The observations lead to the study of genes and behavior.

The **fragile X syndrome** is formed from a peculiar mutated region near the tip of the long arm of the X chromosome. This syndrome is associated with mental retardation. The trinucleotide CGG is present more in the X chromosome and more the copies of the trinucleotide, the more severe is the retardation.

The well studied metabolic error phenylketonuria, also result in mentalpretardation. Similarly the mental deterioration expressed as progressive loss of memory, confusion and anxiety is characteristic of **Alzheimer** disease which has a genetic component. The diagnostic feature of the disease is the deposition of a short protein called beta amyloid, which is derived from a longer protein coded by a gene on chromosome 21. Many other genes are also implicated in Alzheimer disease.

The reading problems collectively known as **dyslexia** also have genetic components. Dyslexic children generally have unexpected problems in learning to read. One form of dyslexia run in families is influenced by a dominant gene located near the centromere of chromosome 15.

Abnormal behaviors are characteristic of Turner syndrome. Down syndrome is also characterized by mental retardation. It is well established that there is a close association between genes and behavior.

### iii. Schizophrenia

Schizophrenia is a behavioral disorder in which the affected person has trouble distinguishing between reality and his or her own imaginings. There is greater variation in the expression of the phenotype. In general schizophrenia is characterized by delusions, illogical response to stimuli, hallucinations, loss of interest in daily life's activities, loss of desire for normal activity and loss of capacity to experience even the simplest of normal pleasures. Nearly 2% of the hospitalized patients are schizophrenics.

Genetic basis of schizophrenia is well established. The study of concordance among MZ twins and DZ twins has given convincing evidence to show the influence of genotype in the development of the disorder. Thirteen studies carried in between 1928 and 1969 indicated the average concordance values to be 52% for 571 pairs of MZ twins and 10% for 1281 pairs of DZ twins. These studies also indicated that while genetical factors are essential for the development of schizophrenia, the environment is also important. A person who has a genotype that predisposes him or her to develop schizophrenia may not express the disorder unless certain environmental factors are present.

There are several models to explain the mode of inheritance of schizophrenia. One model suggests that the disorder is caused by a single autosomal dominant gene. The genetic data gathered shows a correlation between the degree of genetic relatedness and the proportion of relatives affected with schizophrenia. The pre-schizophrenic behavior is characterized by withdrawn and frightened behavior, underdeveloped defenses, a sense of worthlessness and baby like actions.

A second model explains polygenic inheritance for schizophrenia. According to this model, the genes inherited are responsible for the predisposition of the disorder. The condition will develop into schizophrenia only if environmental stresses are present.

A third model for schizophrenia views schizophrenia due to the interaction of genes, genotype and environment. The genotype produces metabolites that induce schizophrenia. Environmental stresses cause the level of steroid hormones to rise, and induce gene activity. The increased activity of certain genes may raise the levels of enzymes responsible for the formation of chemicals such as dimethyltryptamine (DMT) and mescaline. Usually these chemicals are produced at a low level but at higher levels, they are powerful hallucinogenic agents capable of inducing schizophrenia. The elevated levels of these chemicals result in hyperaroused, confused nervous state, which is the cause of schizophrenia. Monamine oxidase (MAO), is an enzyme which usually inactivates neurotransmitters such as dopamine, may be mutant and it's absence increases the levels of neurotransmitters and schizophrenia results.

### iv. Psychosis

There is a mental disorder known as manic depressive psychosis involving extreme behavior anomalies that occur in regular cycles. There is extreme range of mania to deep depression. Suicide is common in persons who have prolonged depression. There is clear genetic basis for psychosis. The genetic analysis reveals that the concordance rate for MZ twins is 76% and 18% for DZ twins. The pedigree studies reveal that a dominant sex linked gene situated closer to the color blindness gene is the causative factor. But studies of L.R. Weitkamp showed that the gene for psychosis is located in the chromosome 6 and is linked to HLA genes. Manic depressive psychosis is of two kinds. The **bipolar** type shows two extremes, mania and depression. The other type namely **unipolar** involves cycle between normality and depression. The types are inherited independently as data suggests unipolar depressives tend to have unipolar relatives and bipolar tend to have bipolar relatives. These two types are symptomatically and pharmacologically distinct from each other.

## 14.2 QUANTITATIVE TRAIT - INTELLIGENCE

Intelligence is a complex phenotype that develops under the influence of genes and the experiences of life time. Psychologists emphasize that intelligence is abstract reasoning ability, which includes thinking rationally, solving problems, understanding the basics of a complex situation, and responding effectively to a new environments. Some psychologists include other abilities such as musical and artistic talent, physical ability, common sense, insight into oneself, and skill in interpersonal relationships.

Intelligence is a complex trait determined by the genotype and environment. It is a group of related abilities such as:

1. Defining and understanding words
2. Thinking of words rapidly
3. Analyzing mathematical relationships
4. Analyzing spatial relationships
5. Memorizing and recalling information
6. Perceiving similarities and differences among objects
7. Formulating rules, principles or concepts for solving problems or understanding situations

It is suggested that there is innate general reasoning ability, but some mental skills, such as musical ability, verbal ability or quantitative ability can be acquired.

Mental ability was first measured by Galton in 1884. In Paris Alfred Binet and his colleagues devised methodologies in 1904 to establish general intelligence. Psychologists at Stanford University developed the Intelligence Quotient (IQ) test. This measures a person's innate intelligence. The IQ is derived by taking a person's mental age (determined by the test), dividing it by his or her actual age and multiplying it by 100. For example if a 10 year old girl has performed the IQ test like a 15 year old girl then her mental age is 15 and her IQ is 150.

It is generally agreed that intelligence is a polygenic trait and subjected to environmental modification. Studies of twins reveal that MZ twins raised together are more concordant for IQ than either MZ twins raised separately or DZ twins raised together. The lower concordance value for MZ twins raised apart indicates that environmental factors can modify the expression of intelligence. MZ twins separated after birth reveals that the greater the environmental differences between them, the greater the IQ differences. In contrast when MZ twins are separated after birth but grown in similar environments showed little differences in IQ. Further, adoption studies have been conducted where IQ of adopted children were compared with their biological mothers and their adoptive mothers. Invariably, a child's IQ was found to be more closely correlated with the IQ of the biological mother than with the adoptive mother. It is suggested that the environmental effect on intelligence is limited.

The twin studies show that the genotype has more influence than the environment. This is supported by data collected comparing the IQ of persons with different degree of genetic relatedness, ranging from identical twins and unrelated persons.

The study reveals that there is a strong genetic component for intelligence. The correlation coefficients indicate that as genetic relatedness among pairs decreases the correlation coefficient also goes down. In a study, unrelated persons raised together such as two boys (with different biological mothers) adopted into the same family with MZ twins raised together are compared and IQ correlation is worked out. The correlation coefficient for the former is 0.23 and the latter is 0.87. This study strengthens the theory of a strong genetic component to the intelligence trait.

## 14.3 PERSONALITY

The systematic study of genetic influences on personality traits was studied by Thomas Bouchard in 1987. The study was based on twins. The twins have been assembled into four groups and compared. The groups were: Monozygotic twins (MZ) raised together, MZ twins raised apart, Dizygotic twins (DZ) raised together and DZ raised apart. All twins were given series of tests to evaluate such personality traits such as leadership, social closeness and traditionalism. From these studies the researchers have concluded that many different personality traits have sizable genetic components with heritability in the range of about 40 – 60%. On the average, about 50% of observed personality diversity can be due to genetic diversity. Many of the environmental influences that affect the development of personality traits tend to come randomly from outside the home that is non shared environment. Even shared family experiences may be perceived differently by each child. Behavioral geneticists have noted that MZ twins brought up in the same family are not much more alike than MZ twins brought up in different families.

## 14.4 ALCOHOLISM

Alcohol intoxication causes depression of the central nervous system, producing uninhibited behavior, poor judgement, incoordination and blackouts. Long-term alcohol abuse is associated with many degenerative diseases, especially of the liver, stomach, heart and brain. In alcoholic women, during pregnancy alcohol diffuse across placenta producing fetal alcohol syndrome, resulting in physical and mental abnormalities.

There are several factors such as personal, social and cultural factors associated with alcoholism. There are evidences to show that some genetic factors are associated with alcoholism. There are two lines of evidences namely 1. Higher concordance in MZ twins than in DZ twins and 2. Increased risk for children of alcoholics even when adopted into nonalcoholic families. In 1970 studies were done to find out the involvement of genetic component in alcoholism. The result of the study is presented in the following table.

**Table 14.1** Alcoholism among male adoptees

| *Biological parent* | *Number in sample* | *% of adopted alcoholic sons* |
|---|---|---|
| Alcoholic father | 89 | 39.4 |
| Alcoholic mother | 42 | 28.6 |
| Nonalcoholic father | 723 | 13.6 |
| Nonalcoholic mother | 1029 | 15.5 |

The table reveals that when adopted males had an alcoholic biological parent, they were 2.3 times more likely to develop alcoholism than when they had nonalcoholic biological parents.

Specific genes that influence alcoholism have been studied in 1990. The researchers discovered a significant genetic difference between group of 35 alcoholics and a control group of nonalcoholics. The gene on the long arm of chromosome 11, encodes a protein that acts as receptor site for a neurotransmitter. A neurotransmitter is a chemical that is released from the end of the nerve cell which binds to the receptor of the next nerve cell facilitating the conduction of nerve impulse.

The receptor protein identified in this study binds to the neurotransmitter dopamine. This substance is present in the regions of brain involved in pleasure seeking. Using molecular probe techniques, the researchers identified two alleles, **A1** and **A2** of this dopamine receptor gene. The A1 allele was present in 69% of the alcoholics, but in only 20% of the nonalcoholics. The role of these alleles in alcoholism is not well established. Genetic investigations of alcoholism are continuing and might throw light on this serious disease and other neurological disorders.

CHAPTER 15

# Detection of Genetic Diseases

## INTRODUCTION

Recent progress in technology and an enhanced understanding of the structure and function of human genes have provided the opportunity to investigate and diagnose genetic disease at the level of abnormal gene itself. Several methods of recombinant DNA technology that have important application to clinical genetics are given below:

## 15.1 RFLP ANALYSIS (RESTRICTION FRAGMENT LENGTH POLYMORPHISM)

The method (Fig. 16.1) relies on the use of **restriction enzymes** that specifically cut the DNA into shorter ends. There are several hundred restriction enzymes available, and each has a specific DNA recognition sequence. For example, the double strand recognition site of the enzyme Eco RI is

———G AATTC———

———CTTAA G———.

RFLP analysis starts by isolating DNA from any sample like blood, liver, muscle, bone, hair etc. The purified DNA is then cleaved with a restriction enzyme.

Restriction enzymes recognize specific short sequences of bases in DNA and cleave large DNA molecules into fragments differing in length. These DNA fragments can be separated by a procedure known as agarose gel elctrophoresis. DNA fragments migrate through the gel, the largest ones remain near the top and smallest ones move more rapidly and migrate to the bottom. When the electrophoretic separation is complete, the fragments of interest are denatured with heat (separated to single strand). They are then transferred from the gel onto solid nitrocellulose or nylon membrane with **Southern blot** technique. After the fragments have been immobilized, fragments can be individually detected by hybridizing a specific radioactive fragment of DNA, called **probe** complementary to the DNA fragments. This procedure of probing a mixture of DNA restriction fragments to identify one specific fragment or gene is called a southern blot.

### Probing for Sickle-cell Anemia

Digestion of normal human DNA by the restriction enzyme Mst11, produces two bands on a southern blot, however the DNA that contains the sickle-cell mutation has lost the middle site and gives one band in southern blot. It is possible to determine the carriers by **RFLP.** The carriers will exhibit two bands of different length and are heterozygous.

## 15.2 FLOURESCENT IN SITU HYBRIDIZATION (FISH)

Fluorescent in situ hybridization was developed in the late 1980s. FISH result in preparations with brilliantly colored whole chromosomes or chromosome parts. Such **chromosome painting** requires complex mixtures of specially constructed DNA sequences, called probes that are complementary to different chromosome regions, together with a set of fluorescent dyes. Also needed is a special microscope with special optical filters, as well as computer software to analyze the image and convert them into a dazzling multicolored display. Chromosome painting is useful for quickly detecting cells with too many or too few chromosomes, or with other types of chromosomal abnormalities, especially in the cancer cells.

### Preparation of Karyotype

Diseases of chromosomal anomalies can be detected by conventional karyotype preparation. A visual karyotype is prepared by arresting dividing cells at metaphase with Colchicine, spreading the cells on a glass side and staining with Giemsa stain. Various banding procedures could be applied. Traditionally a photographic positive is then made and the chromosomes are cut individually and assembled on a card in pairs in order of size following the rules of classification of human chromosomes.

## 15.3 DIAGNOSIS OF METABOLIC DISORDERS

In born errors result from mutations in genes that is responsible for the production of enzyme. Clinical disorders arise from abnormal accumulation of the substrate and/or deficiency of product. Diagnosis can be accomplished by detection of accumulated substance, enzyme assay or direct detection of gene mutations.

For example in PKU, detection of the substrate phenylalanine is accomplished by bacterial inhibition assay. Heel prick blood samples impregnated onto discs of filter paper are placed on a lawn of mutant bacteria that cannot grow in the absence of supplemental phenylalanine. A halo of bacterial growth surrounding a disc indicates a high concentration of phenylalanine in that sample.

Enzyme assay is done in Tay-sacs disease identification. The hexosaminidase –A deficiency is quantified and carrier could be identified.

DNA diagnosis by RFLP, FISH etc is increasingly being used as a direct approach to diagnosis of inborn errors of metabolism.

## 15.4 POLYMERASE CHAIN REACTION (PCR)

It is a powerful technique for selective and rapid amplification of target DNA or RNA sequences. The technique is based on the enzymatic amplification of a DNA fragment that is flanked by two stretches of nucleotide primers, which hybridize to opposite strands of the sequence being investigated.

This technique works by using heat to separate the two strands of DNA, which allows primers to bind to their complementary sequence. The segment between the primers is amplified in the presence of Taq polymerase enzyme and deoxynucleotides. The amount of amplified DNA increases rapidly each time the cycle occurs. Repetition of the cycle can produce millions of copies of the DNA under investigation.

PCR is extremely valuable because of the speed, sensitivity and requirement of minute quantity of sample.

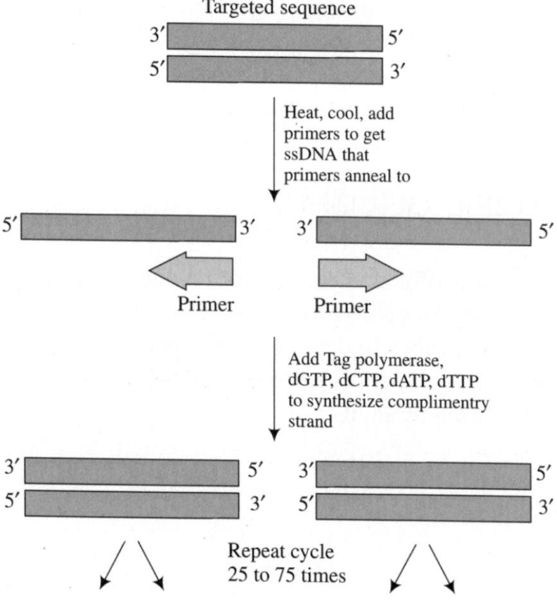


**Fig. 15.1** Polymerase chain reaction
(Source : www.microbeworld.com)

### PCR-single-strand Conformation Polymorphism (PCR-SSCP)

Many inherited disorders are due to single nucleotide changes within critical regions of the affected gene (e.g. Sickle cell anemia). The PCR-SSCP technique can detect single mutations in genes due to the altered mobility of the single strands of DNA (in electrophoresis) carrying the mutant compared to the wild type. Specific primers are made for the sequences of a disease gene where a mutation is known to exist and the region is amplified by PCR. The same region of the wild type gene is amplified by PCR. The two strands of mutant PCR product will migrate differently than the two strands of the wild type PCR product. Even single mutations can be detected by observing the amplified DNA having different mobility due to altered conformations when subjected to electrophoresis in non-denaturing gels.

The PCR products following gel electrophoresis can be visualized clearly by either using radioactively labeled primers or incorporating radioactive nucleotides into PCR products. The PCR products are separated in a polyacrylamide gel and observed by exposing the gel to X-ray film. Individuals that are homozygous wild-type or mutant homozygous will show two bands in the gel. However the mutant PCR products will migrate with different mobilities in the gel. Individuals that are heterozygous will exhibit a pattern consisting of all four bands.

### The Ligase Chain Reaction (LCR)

The LCR is another technique that detects single point mutations in a disease gene. The technique employs a thermostable DNA ligase to ligate adjacent oligonucleotides. Two sets of oligonucleotides are designed to anneal to one strand of the gene at the site of the mutation, a second set of two oligonucleotides anneal to the other strand. The oligonucleotides are prepared in such a way that they will anneal completely with the wild type sequences only. For example in sickle cell mutation, the 3' nucleotide of one oligonucleotide in each pair is mismatched. This mismatch prevents the annealing of the oligonucleotide directly adjacent to each other. Therefore, DNA ligase will not ligate the two oligonucleoties of each pair together. The oligonucleotides that are ligated together anneal and result in exponential amplification of the wild type.

## 15.5 ALLELE SPECIFIC OLIGONUCLEOTIDE (ASO) PROBE ANALYSIS

This technique uses two synthetic oligonucleotide probes: one probe specific for a normal gene and the other probe specific for a known genetic mutation. The ASO probes for the normal and mutant genes are used as hybridization probes to determine whether a patient has two copies of a normal gene or a mutation responsible for a particular disease. ASO probe analysis can be used on DNA that has been selectively amplified by PCR.

CHAPTER 16

# DNA Fingerprinting

## INTRODUCTION

Personal identification involves a standard method of analyzing, a persons fingerprints. Constant throughout life, fingerprint ridge patterns can be used to distinguish one person from any other, even identical twins, although their patterns are very similar.

DNA fingerprinting has a similar aim, but it is based on certain nucleotide sequences that differ greatly among people. (This is rightly called **DNA profiling** or **DNA typing**, since it has nothing to do with fingers). Alec Jeffrey of Leicester University, England developed this technique in 1983.

DNA fingerprinting was first used in England in 1986 to prosecute a rape-murder trial. DNA from sperm found on the victims genitals was compared with DNA from white blood cells of possible suspects.

## 16.1 PRINCIPLE

The genetic material of the human being (genome) consists of 3 billion nucleotides ($3 \times 10^9$). Encoded in this DNA is the information for about 30,000 genes. About 95% of the DNA is considered "junk", that is, it may not have a known function and is the non coding region of DNA. About 5% of the DNA has a known function and is considered the coding regions of the DNA. The non coding region has more sequence variation. DNA profiling makes use of the coding as well as the non coding regions.

There are many places in human DNA where sequences of nucleotides are repeated over and over. For example, there is a particular sequence in human DNA which is 16 nucleotides long.

AGAGGTGGGCAGGTGG

This sequence is repeated hundreds of times in different regions of chromosomes. These repetitive regions do not code for polypeptides. They are just present there. No two people are likely to have the same number of copies of these. These regions are called **VNTRS**, which stands for variable number of tandem repeats. The number of repetitive regions and hence the size of the VNTRs, varies markedly between individuals, and is inherited: half of the repeats derive from the father and the other half from the mother. Only identical twins have the same numbers of repeats.

The degree of variation in bands from one person to another is so large that the theoretical probability that the bands seen in one individual are present in another unrelated individual may be one in many millions or billions. Essentially, each person has a unique DNA fingerprint.

## 16.2 THE SEQUENCE OF EVENTS IN DNA FINGERPRINTING

Let us assume that two DNA samples are at hand, one from blood spots found at the scene of a crime and another from a suspect.

The analysis proceeds as follows:

1. The two DNA samples from the blood samples are treated separately with restriction enzyme such as EcoRI, which cuts DNA at all GAATTC sites. When it cuts, the pieces may include the **VNTR** regions of varying length. The fragments generated, vary from one person to another. The EcoRI generate 100,000 pieces of varying sizes, a few of which include the VNTR regions.
2. Electrophoresis is used to spread out the 100,000 fragments, or bands, of DNA according to size. The two samples are run in side-by-side lanes along with control lanes containing DNA segments of known size.
3. The pattern of DNA bands in the gel is transferred to a nylon membrane. This is accomplished by laying the membrane on top of the gel and setting DNA diffuse up from gel. This is southern blotting. The liquid that moves up through the gel and membrane also denatures the DNA, so single-stranded DNA stick to the membrane corresponding to the bands in the gel.
4. The nylon membrane is removed and incubated with radioactive probe, which is single-stranded DNA complementary to the repetitive DNA. This probe hybridizes with complimentary DNA sequences wherever they occur in the nylon membrane.
5. The final step is autoradiography. A sheet of x-ray film is laid on the membrane, and bands appear wherever the radioactive rays from probe sensitizes the film. Dark bands appear in the film representing the various length of DNA discovered by the probe.

The probe which detects many different regions is called a **multi locus probe.** On the contrary, a **single locus probe** will hybridize to just one VNTR region in an individual's DNA giving a genetic finger print of two bands for an individual, one from the maternal, and one from the

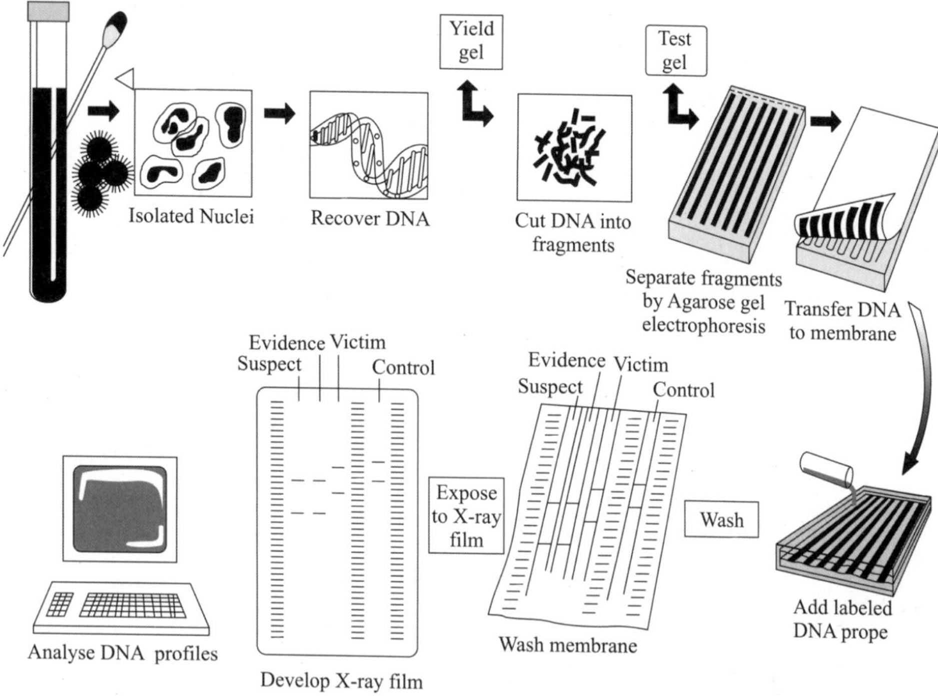


**Fig. 16.1** DNA fingerprinting
(Source : www.freeweb.com)

paternal. Single locus probes are more sensitive than multi locus probes. In forensic work, several single locus probes are used on a single sample.

### PCR-Based Method

This is the most sensitive methods which utilizes polymerase chain reaction. Here a specific polymorphic gene is amplified by cyclic reaction using PCR. The various genes that are present in the biological samples are revealed by using a set of specific probes. The hybridization of these alleles to their probes is revealed by a dye (often a fluorescent stain) that binds only to double stranded DNA. Electrophoresis, blotting and radioactivity are not needed. This is a simplified method. The major advantage is that it needs less than 1 microgram of DNA and can be performed quickly.

## 16.3 APPLICATIONS

- DNA fingerprinting is widely applied in court proceedings to establish family relationships in disputed parentage. DNA fingerprints of the child can be compared with those of putative parents and with other family members to establish positive relationship.
- DNA fingerprinting can be applied in forensic science in identifying the criminals.

- In determining species variation to establish biodiversity, gene banking and genetic screening of animals and plants.
- In identifying the pure breed for selective breeding in animal breeding programs.
- Tracking the illegal trading of endangered wild animals.
- In confirming the microbial strain in contaminated food stuff.
- Confirming animal pedigrees.

CHAPTER 17

# Human Gene Mapping

## INTRODUCTION

Genetic linkage is the tendency for alleles close together on the same chromosome to be transmitted together to offspring. It is of great value in genetic prognosis. Disease association is the appearance in many patients of a genetically determined character at a frequency higher than that would predicted on the basis of their independent frequencies. A group of disease features that regularly occur together, usually due to pleiotropic expression of one allele is called a syndrome.

In order to know about the details of a genetic disease, it is important to identify the position of the gene responsible for the disease in the chromosome. The first step therefore is locating the position of a particular gene among other genes along a chromosome. There are different ways of determining the position of a gene in the chromosome.

## 17.1 GENETIC LINKAGE MAPPING

Gene mapping often begins with a statistical analysis of the consequences of crossing over during meiosis in successive generations. The analysis of crossing over leads to the construction of **genetic linkage maps**.

Assume two loci, **A** and **B** are close together on the same chromosome and the mating types could be type (i) **AB//ab** × **ab//ab** or type (ii) **Ab//**aB × **ab//ab**, where/represents a chromosome. In type (i) matings, dominant alleles **A** and **B** are on the same chromosome and recessive alleles **a** and **b** on its homologous chromosome. The dominants and recessives are said to be 'in coupling', or **cis** to one another. In mating type (ii) the dominant and recessive alleles on opposite chromosomes are 'in repulsion', or trans to one another.

Since loci **A** and **B** are close crossing over rarely occur between them and the parental combinations **AB** and **ab** or **Ab** and **aB**, will be more frequently represented among offspring than the recombinant combinations **Ab** and **aB** or **AB** and **ab** respectively.

If an allele of gene A causes disease, but is otherwise undetectable, whereas the alleles of gene B can be easily detected and distinguished, gene B can be used as a marker for the inherited disease.

The genetic map distance between loci A and B can be deduced from the frequency of recombination between them by the formula:

Number of recombinant offspring × 100 / Total number offspring

In type (i) matings: (Aabb + aaBb) × 100/ Aabb + aaBb + AaBb + aabb

In type (ii) matings: ( AaBb + aabb) × 100 / Aabb + aaBb + AaBb + aabb

The unit of map distance (the distance between genes) is **centiMorgan (cM)** and is termed **map unit**.

X map unit = X % recombination

A 1% recombination is interpreted as 1 map unit, 5% recombination as 5 map units, and so on.

The total map length of the genome, estimated from crossing over in primary germ cells is - 3000cM in males and –4200cM in females.

The reliability of a suspected linkage can be confirmed by **'LOD score analysis'** of family pedigrees. The word LOD is derived from 'log of odds', the logarithm ($\log_{10}$) of the ratio of the probability that the observed ratio of offspring arose as result of genetic linkage to the probability that it arose merely by chance.

## 17.2 DNA MARKER MAPS

DNA markers have proved very useful in linkage studies, and about 10,000 such sites have been positioned on the Human chromosomes. The first DNA markers that were extensively used are called RFLPs. Others are microsatellites, very short units repeated 20 to 30 times, and VNTRs, somewhat longer repeats that are basis of some DNA fingerprinting.

Restriction fragment length polymorphism is based on substitution mutations that alter the recognition sites of restriction enzymes. Thus, at those particular spots, the enzyme cuts one person's DNA but not another's. For example, suppose that in one person's DNA there are four for E.coli restriction enzyme EcoRI spaced as follows:

—X——————X——X——————X———

7kb 1kb 4kb

Whereas the same section in another person's DNA has only three EcoRI sites

—X————————————X——————X———

8kb 4kb

The difference is due to mutations and most of them are not in protein encoding genes. The variations they produce can be detected by the technique described for DNA fingerprinting in the previous chapter.

**Huntington disease** was the first disease – producing gene mapped by DNA markers. The gene was located to an RFLP site about 4 map units away near the tip of the short arm of chromosome 4. Later researchers found DNA markers within 1 or 2 map units on both sides of the gene. These are called flanking markers. Similarly the breast cancer gene BRCA1 is within 10 map units of a VNTR with multiple alleles in band q21 of chromosome 17.

The frequency of cross over is near the ends of the chromosomes. On the average, the approximately $3 \times 10^9$ base pairs of a haploid genome are divided into 3,700 units for all human chromosomes. Thus $(3 \times 10^9) / 3{,}700$, or approximately 800,000 base pairs, correspond to 1 map unit. So if a disease gene is flanked by known DNA markers, each 1.25 map units away, the gene resides in a DNA interval of 2 million base pairs.

## 17.3 PHYSICAL MAPS

Physical maps are based on cytological landmarks on the chromosomes like rearrangements, duplications etc. Physical mapping deals with sequencing lengths of DNA by ordering individual bases A, T, G and C.

The technique called **somatic cell fusion** is applied in cytological mapping. The laboratory cultured human cells and mouse cells are fused to form hybrid cells by the fusion agents like PEG or Sendai virus. In such hybrid cells it is interesting to note that all the mouse chromosomes remain while some human chromosomes are lost. The reason for preferential loss is not clear. Which particular human chromosomes are lost and which ones are retained seems to be random. Based on this sub clones could be produced.

The loss of the chromosome is often accompanied by loss of a protein encoded by the gene. By associating the gene product with the chromosome the location of the gene can be predicted. For example the enzyme Thymidine kinase is absent in the cells where the chromosome 17 is lost or whenever the cell contains chromosome 17, the Thymidine kinase enzyme is always present.

Another method for gene localization is **FISH** (introduced in Chapter 7). In this technique first human metaphase chromosomes are prepared. After removing RNA and proteins single stranded DNA are produced. These DNA are bathed with a single stranded probe specific for a given gene. This probe is chemically linked to fluorochrome, a molecule that illuminates under UV rays. Using different fluorochromes multiple coloured chromosomes could be displayed. Thus the chromosomes are painted and could be labeled with a specific gene sequence. By FISH technique spatial organization of the genes could be observed.

### Ordered DNA Segments

Finer physical mapping involve cloning segments of DNA and arranging the segments in order. The collection of cloned segments can span a region that is cut with a restriction enzyme or a region between two DNA markers (whose linkage distance has been established by FISH) Such a collection of fragments is called a **contig**, short for "contiguous set of cloned segments".

Yeast artificial chromosomes (YAC) is used to clone the DNA segment from the human chromosome. If the human DNA is about 500kb long then YAC is used. Bacterial artificial chromosome (BAC) can be used if the inserts are about 150kb. Phage artificial chromosome (PAC) can contain inserts of about 100kb, and cosmids are preferred for some application like when the DNA segment is about 40kb long. Construction of a contig of overlapping clones with a overlapping DNA pieces are utilized in this technique.

The method of choice to align and order a set of YACs, BACs, PACs or cosmids involves sequencing just short randomly selected segments of the cloned human DNA. These sites are called **sequence tagged sites (STSs)**, and each is about 200 nucleotides long. By publishing 20-base sequences toward the ends of STSs, researchers make it possible for any laboratory in the world to reproduce the STSs in their own DNA samples by the Polymerase chain reaction, using the published sequences as primers. An STS-based map of almost the entire human genome has been assembled. This map includes about 15,000 STSs whose positions are anchored by known genetic linkages. The STS map is a key tool for identifying disease genes.

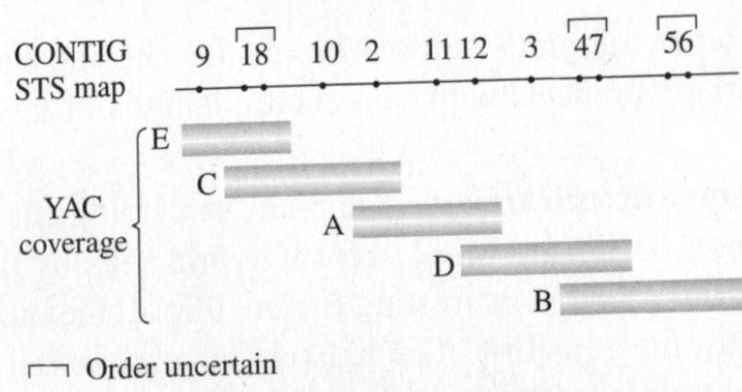


**Fig. 17.1** Contig construction using YAC
(Source : www.nature.com)

## Base Sequence Data

The ultimate physical map of human DNA is the specification of base-by-base determination using the common Sanger method. The human DNA insert (10,000 to 40,000 bases) in a plasmid, phage or artificial chromosome by first breaking up the DNA into overlapping 300 to 500-base pieces and order them by the overlapping regions. Advances in computer-base methods for collecting, storing, distributing and analyzing are also done in automated **DNA Sequencer**.

It is known that the cDNA, without introns includes only genes that are expressed. J.Craig Venter analyzed the cDNA molecules obtained from the mRNAs isolated from dozens of different human organs and tissues. But instead of sequencing the several kilobases of each cDNA, he sequenced only a few hundred bases from each cDNA molecule. These segments are called **expressed sequence tags (ESTs)**, that is, markers for genes that are expressed in a particular tissue.

CHAPTER 18

# Human Genome Project

## INTRODUCTION

The U.S. Human Genome Project (**HGP**) was begun formally in 1990, a 13 years effort coordinated by the U.S. Department of Energy and the National Institutes of Health. In 1997, United States established the National Human Genome Research Institute (NHGRI). The HGP was an international venture involving countries like USA, UK, France, Germany, Japan and China. The project originally was planned to last 15 years, but rapid technological advances accelerated the completion date to 2003. On 26$^{th}$ June 2000 Francis Collins and Craig Venter announced the first draft of human genome sequence.

## 18.1 PROJECT GOALS

- identify all the approximate 30,000 genes in human DNA,
- determine the sequences of the 3 billion chemical base pairs that make up human DNA,
- store this information in databases,
- improve tools for data analysis,
- transfer related technologies to the private sector and
- address the ethical, legal, and social issues (**ELSI**) that may arise from the project.

To help achieve these goals, researchers also studied the genetic makeup of several nonhuman organisms. These include the common human gut bacterium Escherichia coli, the fruit fly, and the laboratory mouse.

- A **genome** is the total DNA in an organism, including its genes. Genes carry information for making all the proteins required by all organisms. These proteins determine, among other things, how the organism looks, how well its body metabolizes food or fights infection, and sometimes even how it behaves.
- DNA is made up of four similar chemicals (called bases and abbreviated A, T, C and G) that are repeated millions or billions of times throughout a genome. The human genome for example, has 3 billion pairs of bases.
- The particular order of As, Ts, Cs and Gs is extremely important. The order underlies all of life's diversity, even dictating whether an organism is human or another species such as yeast, rice, or fruit fly, all of which have their own genomes and are themselves the focus of genome projects. Because all organisms are related through similarities in DNA sequences, insights gained from nonhuman genomes often lead to new knowledge about human biology.

## 18.2 STEPS INVOLVED IN HGP

There are various techniques used to sequence the human DNA. These techniques include:

- The Employment of Restriction Fragment-Length Polymorphisms (**RFLP**)
- Yeast Artificial Chromosomes **(YAC)**
- Bacterial Artificial Chromosomes **(BAC)**
- The Polymerase Chain Reaction **(PCR)**
- Electrophoresis

A sample of widely used technique is as follows:

### Bacterial Artificial Chromosomes (BAC)

Sequencing means determining the exact order of the base pairs in a segment of DNA. Human chromosomes range in size, from about 50,000,000 to 300, 000, 000 base pairs. Because the bases exist as pairs, and the identity of one of the bases in the pair determines the other member of the pair, scientists do not have to report both bases of the pair.

The primary method used by the HGP to produce the finished version of the human genetic code is map based, or BAC-based sequencing. BAC is the acronym for "bacterial artificial chromosome." Human DNA is fragmented into pieces that are relatively large but still manageable in size (between 150, 000 and 200,000 base pairs). The fragments are cloned in bacteria, which store and replicate the human DNA so that it can be prepared in quantities large enough for sequencing. If carefully chosen to minimize overlap, it takes about 20,000 different BAC clones to contain the 3 billion pairs of bases of the human genome. A collection of BAC clones containing the entire human genome is called a **"BAC library."**

In the BAC-based method, each BAC clone is "mapped" to determine where the DNA in BAC clones comes from in the human genome. Using this approach ensures that scientists know both the precise location of the DNA letters that are sequenced from each clone and their spatial relation to sequenced human DNA in BAC clones.

For sequencing, each BAC clone is cut into still smaller fragments that are about 2,000 bases in length. These pieces are called "subclones." A "sequencing reaction" is carried out on these subclones. The products of the sequencing reaction are then loaded into the sequencing machine (sequencer). The sequencer generates about 500 to 800 base pairs of A, T, C and G from each sequencing reaction, so that each base is sequenced about 10 times. A computer then assembles these short sequences into contiguous stretches of sequence representing the human DNA in the BAC clone.

## 18.3 MILESTONES IN HGP

On June 26, 2000, the International Human Genome Sequencing Consortium announced the production of a rough draft of the human genome sequence. In April, 2003, the International Human Genome Sequencing announced an essentially finished version of the human genome sequence.

### a. By Numbers

- The human genome contains 3164.7 million chemical nucleotide bases (A, C, T and G).
- The actual part of the genome that codes for proteins makes up less than 2% while repeated sequences make up at least 50%. The repeats have no direct function but they shed light on chromosome structure and dynamics.
- The average gene consists of 3000 bases, but sizes vary greatly, with the largest known human gene being dystrophin at 2.4 million bases.
- The total number of genes is estimated at 30,000-much lower than previous estimates of 80,000 to 140,000.
- Almost all (99.9%) nucleotide bases are exactly the same in all people.
- Chromosome 1 has the most genes (2968), and the Y chromosome has the fewest (231).

### b. By Arrangement

- The human genome's gene-dense "urban centers" are pre-dominantly composed of the DNA building blocks G and C.
- In contrast, the gene-poor "deserts" are rich in the DNA building blocks A and T. GC-and AT-rich regions usually can be seen through a microscope as light and dark bands on chromosomes.
- Genes appear to be concentrated in random areas along the genome, with vast expanses of non-coding DNA between.
- Stretches of up to 30,000 C and G bases repeating over and over often occur adjacent to gene-rich areas, forming a barrier between the genes and the "junk DNA". The vast majority (45%) of repeated sequences in the human genome are derived from transposons.

## 18.4 SOME CHROMOSOMES AND THEIR GENES

### Chromosome 22

Chromosome 22 is the first of 23 human chromosome pairs to be deciphered because of its relatively small size and its association with several diseases. A total number of at least 545 genes and 134 pseudogenes (genes that once functioned but no longer do) were detected on the chromosome. The genes range in size from 1,000 to 583,000 bases of DNA with a mean size of 190,000 bases. Sequencing and mapping efforts have revealed that chromosome 22 is implicated in the workings of the immune system, congenital heart disease, schizophrenia, mental retardation, birth defects, and several cancers including leukemia.

### Chromosome 7

Chromosome 7 was the focus of much attention from geneticists during the search for the Cystic fibrosis gene (CFTR). Other diseases linked with this chromosome include, Retinosis pigmentosa, and cancers including Wilm's tumour.

## 18.5 CURRENT AND POTENTIAL APPLICATIONS OF GENOME RESEARCH

### i. Molecular Medicine

- improved diagnosis of disease
- earlier detection of genetic predispositions to disease
- rational drug design and pharmacogenomics
- gene therapy and control systems for drugs

### ii. Risk Assessment

- assess health damage and risks caused by radiation exposure, including low-dose exposures
- assess health damage and risks caused by exposure to mutagenic chemicals and cancer-causing toxins
- reduce the likelihood of heritable mutations

### iii Anthropology, Evolution, and Human Migration

- study evolution through germ line mutations in lineages
- study migration of different population groups based on female genetic inheritance
- study mutations on the Y chromosome to trace lineage and migration of males
- compare breakpoints in the evolution of mutations with ages of populations and historical events

### iv. DNA Forensics and Identification

- identify potential suspects whose DNA may match evidence left at crime scenes
- exonerate persons wrongly accused of crimes
- identify crime and catastrophe victims
- establish paternity and other family relationships
- detect bacteria and other organisms that may pollute air, water, soil and food
- match organ donors with recipients in transplant programs

## 18.6 FUTURE CHALLENGES

The human genome is as complete as it can be with the available technology. Small gaps remain, amounting for about 1 percent of the gene-containing portion of the genome. New technologies will have to be invented to obtain the sequence of these regions. However, the gene-containing portion of the genome is complete in nearly every functional way for the purposes of scientific research and is freely and publicly available. NHGRI has proposals to support a wide range of research to develop new sequencing technologies, to interpret the human sequence and to use the newfound understanding of the human genome to improve human health.

The knowledge derived from the DNA sequence will define research through the coming decades to inform our understanding of biological systems. This enormous task will require the expertise and creativity of tens of thousands of scientists from varied disciplines in both the public and private sectors worldwide.

A number of genes have been pinpointed and associated with breast cancer, muscle disease, deafness, and blindness. Additionally, finding the DNA sequences underlying such common diseases as cardiovascular disease, diabetes, arthritis, and cancers can promote the development of effective new therapies.

In the past, researchers studied one or a few genes at a time. With whole-genome sequences, they can study all the genes in a genome. For example, all the transcripts in a particular tissue or organ or tumor, or how thousand of genes and proteins work together in interconnected networks to orchestrate the chemistry of life can be revealed.

But there has been controversy. Some say that the technical knowledge has outpaced the ability to handle the social implications. Test can be done for ills that can not be treated. A fetus for Down syndrome can be tested, but it is not possible to determine whether the child will be mildly or severely affected. There are genes involved in personality traits, but the implications of telling a person that he or she is "predisposed" to, say, anxiety may complicate things. Genetics show that the racial distinctions made between people are cultural, not biological-so what does it mean to say that more African-Americans have sickle cell, or that more Euro-Americans have cystic fibrosis? So, even after all these developments there are issues to be discussed and discovered.

## 18.7 ETHICAL, LEGAL AND SOCIAL IMPLICATION (ELSI) OF HGP

James Watson, the first director of human genome research in the National Institute of Health, established a group to investigate the ethical, legal and social implications of the HGP. The ELSI group consists of medical geneticists, ethicists, theologians, lawyers, social scientists, and others with special expertise. It receives 3-5% of the annual budget of the HGP to support public conferences, workshops, special commissions and research proposals. Areas of study include the use of genetic testing in clinical practice, the access to genetic information to any body and the understanding of the power and limitations of genetics by the public. Maintaining confidentiality of medical data is another area of concern.

The following questions have to be answered in dealing with HGP:

- Can the genetic information of a person be kept confidential?
- Will the DNA sample be stored for future use or destroyed when the person dies?
- Will the DNA sample used for research without the person's consent?
- Will the patient be given full detail about his genes?
- Will the information gained through DNA testing and analyses revealed to the family members?

The main problem will be cloning of the specific gene and the identification of mutation that causes the disease permitting the commercial exploitation of genetic tests. For example Myriad Genetics and other companies have introduced commercial testing for mutations in the BRCAI gene that lead to breast cancer in about 85% of cases and to ovarian cancer in about 45% of cases. Critics of marketing the BRCAI test emphasize the need for expert counseling to help patients and their families decide on testing, interpret the results and face uncertainty.

A woman at risk may have multitude of questions; is the test 100% accurate? Dose the presence of a mutant allele mean certain breast or ovarian cancer? At what age? What are the options? Will surgery reduce the cancer risk to zero? What about my sister and daughter? What effect it will have on my employment? Can I hide the results under a false name or a code?

CHAPTER 19

# Genetic Counseling

## INTRODUCTION

The incidence of human diseases have decreased by modern medicine and effective community health measures. There is increase in awareness of genetic diseases. Genetic counseling deals with the problem of giving advice to families, having or likely to have children with genetic disorders.

The aim of genetic counseling is to convey medical and genetic facts to an affected family in a way that can be understood. Genetic counseling is relatively a new area of human genetics and many are not aware of its existence. Genetic counseling requires professionals who have good knowledge in both genetics and medicine. To this must be added patience, sensitivity, respect and the ability to talk easily with people who are likely to be troubled. The affected family must be helped to have decisions they are comfortable with. These families must be provided with a full range of medical and social services.

Every year thousands of families are affected by the birth of an abnormal child. About 0.7% of newborns have a chromosomal abnormality, another 1% suffers single gene defects and about 2% have malformations, putting altogether, about 4% newborns have a defect.

Our knowledge of genetics permits relatively accurate prediction, based on statistical probability, of the recurrence of genetic defects and diseases within families. With proper genetic counseling, the appearance of serious, sometimes fatal diseases can be avoided by preventing the conception of sick human being. A voluntary restriction of child bearing by couples who carry serious hereditary defects can be brought about through proper genetic counseling. Such voluntary restriction would reduce the transmission of many hereditary abnormalities when the information is available.

The purpose of genetic counseling is to prevent the misery imposed on the individual as well as his family through the birth of defective children. Such counseling help to reduce the number of genetically affected families and thus, in the population at large and therefore could be enforcing eugenics.

## 19.1 INDICATIONS FOR GENETIC COUNSELING

1. Advanced maternal age
2. Known or suspected hereditary condition in the family
3. Consanguinity
4. Recurrent spontaneous abortions
5. A fetus or child with birth defects
6. Exposure to known teratogens

## 19.2 GENETIC COUNSELING TEAM

Genetic counseling is a communication process which deals with human problems associated with the occurrence, or the risk of occurrence of a genetic disorder in a family. This process involves an attempt by one or more appropriately trained persons (genetic counseling) to help the individual or family to

(i) comprehend the medical facts, including the diagnosis, the probable course of the disorder, and the available management
(ii) appreciate the way heredity contributes to disorder, and the risk of recurrence in specified relatives
(iii) understand the options for dealing with the risk of recurrence
(iv) choose the course of action which seems appropriate to them in view of their risk and the family goals and in accordance with the decision
(v) make the best possible adjustment to the disorder in the affected family member and/or the risk of recurrence of that disorder

Genetic counseling is effectively done by a team comprising

i. The medical specialist is trained in medical speciality and is a medical practitioner. He plays a consultant role.
ii. The genetic counselor is a trained person in counseling with a sound knowledge in Human Genetics. The role of the counselor is to be involved in the counseling process, support and follow-up of the family.
iii. Additional members may be included like social workers, religious support persons and family physicians

## 19.3 TYPES OF GENETIC COUNSELING

In general there are two ways by which genetic counseling is effected. They are **prospective counseling** and **retrospective counseling**. Prospective counseling is delivered to a person in the reproductive age group before the birth of an affected child. On the other hand retrospective counseling is rendered after the birth of an affected child. In practice most of the counseling is retrospective and a majority of those having an afflicted child still probably do not receive genetic counseling due to paucity of genetic counseling centers. There are many advantages in prospective counseling. This would permit decisions to be made whether pregnancy should be undertaken and whether prenatal diagnosis would be useful. Moreover, early recognition of genetic disorders, which are preventable or treatable, is desirable.

## 19.4 THE PROCESS

The following are the various steps required for any form of genetic counseling:

Step I - Determining the risk.

Step II - Interpretation and communication of the recurrence risk.

Step III - Formulation of a rational approach.

Step IV - Follow-up.

### a. Medical Diagnosis

Precise diagnosis is required as many hereditary diseases have multiple causes. Some diseases are phenotypically indistinguishable from one another. The propositus is first examined and in addition other family members are examined. Laboratory work often includes karyotyping; biochemical analyses of blood, urine or cultured cells; or molecular analysis with restriction enzymes and DNA probes. The work involved in corresponding with relatives and autopsy report is very time consuming and tedious. A correct diagnosis is the corer stone of useful genetic counseling since a wrong diagnosis often have dangerous consequences.

### b. Pedigree Analysis

A complete three to four generation family pedigree must be obtained and analyzed. The reliability of the collected information must be thoroughly assessed. Some important clues-adoptions, illegitimate births, miscarriages, still births or mildly affected relatives may be entirely missing. Thus decision on the inheritance pattern of the disease must be made analyzing all the facts. Pedigree analysis has been already discussed in chapter 4.

### c. Estimating Recurrence Risks

The answer to the question, how likely is it that a disease will recur in a subsequent birth? is straight forward.

If it is an autosomal recessive allele then the probability is 25% when the parents are known to be heterozygous. The probability of having an affected child is the product of the probabilities of parents being carrier, multiplied by 1/4, i.e., if two cousins of an affected individual marry each other the risk of each child of theirs being affected is 1/4 × 1/4 × 1/4 or 1 in 64.

For a person heterozygous for an autosomal dominant allele, the chances of any of his children being affected are 50%.

In an X-linked trait, the sister of an affected male(because of their mother being a carrier) has 50% chances of being a carrier and therefore the chances of any of her sons being affected are 1in 4. If a woman has only one son affected, it can be due to a mutation.

With the advancement in DNA technology, more and more disease causing Mendelian genes can be analyzed prenatally using fetal cells obtained by different techniques discussed in the next chapter. Direct detection of a disease-causing allele can also be done in some cases by using DNA probes.

Counselors cannot establish a risk figure based on rules of transmission if the disease is caused by multiple factors. In these cases, counselor can make use of **empiric risk** figures that rely on the statistics of prior experience with the particular disease in question. For many congenital malformations, such as spina bifida, cleft lip or club foot, the risk of recurrence of the particular malformation after the birth of one affected child to normal parents is about 2-5%. For certain traits, the geographical or racial background of a couple may be an important element of risk estimation.

For Down syndrome, it is important to distinguish between a non-disjunctional cause and the presence of a translocation. Most cases of Down syndrome are due to non-disjunction, and the risk of recurrence is small. Less often, Down syndrome is due to a translocation in a parent, and the risk of recurrence is relatively high.

Even if there is no family history of Down syndrome, there are sporadic risks that increase with advancing maternal age. It is an established fact that as a woman gets older, the chance that she may have an abnormal pregnancy involving an extra or missing chromosome increases. Women's egg cells are in their bodies from the time they are born. If a woman is 20 years of age, her egg cells are also 20 years old. If a woman is 40 years old, her egg cells are also 40. Sperm cells are newly made every day and have fewer aging issues. Down syndrome and other chromosome abnormalities may happen at any age, but increase each year along with a woman's age. The following table indicates the maternal age effect.

**Table 19.1** Maternal age and Birth rates for children with chromosomal abnormalities – Approximate risks

| *Maternal Age* | *Risk* |
|---|---|
| 20 | 1 in 525 |
| 25 | 1 in 475 |
| 30 | 1 in 380 |
| 36 | 1 in 180 |
| 38 | 1 in 105 |
| 40 | 1 in 65 |
| 42 | 1 in 40 |
| 45 | 1 in 20 |

The risk figures must be conveyed in such a manner that they can be understood. Repeating information in different ways may be useful. The risk of recurrence for a simple Mendelian trait is the same for each birth, regardless of prior outcomes. For example, if unaffected carrier parents produce one child with a recessive disorder, this does not mean that the next three children will be normal. The risk of an affected child on each successive birth continues to be 1/4.

## 19.5 OPTIONS

A couple may refrain from childbearing risk a defective birth, when the genetic prognosis is unfavorable. If abortion is an acceptable alternative, prenatal diagnosis (followed by termination of pregnancy) is now available for a number of cases. Alternatively a couple may choose adoption or an appropriate reproductive technology like IVF (in vitro fertilization) using donor sperm or donor egg.

One's perception of risk and willingness to accept it depend on one's moral convictions, experiences and especially on the burden of care that the family has to take up. Some newborns with birth defects may die within few months. Some may require constant attention from their family throughout their life and may require expensive medical treatment.

A couple may need time to talk it out between themselves and with friends and relatives, the process should not be hurried. So the humanistic aspects of counseling are extremely important. Decision making may be difficult in most of the cases. The counselor must understand and help a mother who blames herself for bearing a child with birth defect or a father who may deny the child is his biological offspring.

## 19.6 FOLLOW-UP AND SUPPORTIVE SERVICES

The relevant medical and genetic information must be put in writing as there is a possibility for the counselor's words to be mistaken or forgotten. Families should be informed of useful new research results and be allowed to decide on participating in experimental trials. Services can also be extended to relatives who may unknowingly be at risk. A counselor must provide expert and caring assistance to persons whose self-esteem has been hurt and whose lives have become complicated suddenly by the birth of a child with genetic disorder.

For various genetic diseases support groups have been established at the local, regional, national and international levels. These organizations take up issues on genetic diseases or publish educational material to help laypersons as well as professionals. However, their greatest value is in peer support, demonstrating to families affected by a genetic disease that they are not alone, that they can share their burden, frustration and doubts. There are over 300 of these groups belonging to 'Alliance of Genetic support groups' based in Washington is available to take up supportive service.

## 19.7 GENETIC SCREENING

Genetic counseling is essentially a communication process that gives information to the prospective parents about the risk of having a genetically defective child, about the nature of the genetic disorders and the options available to them in dealing with that risk. Or it can help them cope with the care of an existing genetically handicapped child.

In contrast, **genetic screening**, is a routine diagnostic procedure employed to detect those are affected by a hereditary disease or carriers of defective gene. Genetic screening applies to population than to individual.

For example the most-widespread application of genetic screening in USA is for phenylketonuria (PKU). All hospitals in the USA screen newborn for PKU by a blood test called Guthrie test. A drop of the infant's blood is checked for the presence of excess of phenylalanine, one of the twenty amino acids. If a PKU infant is detected, the effects of the disease can be prevented by providing a diet with a low phenylalanine to the infant.

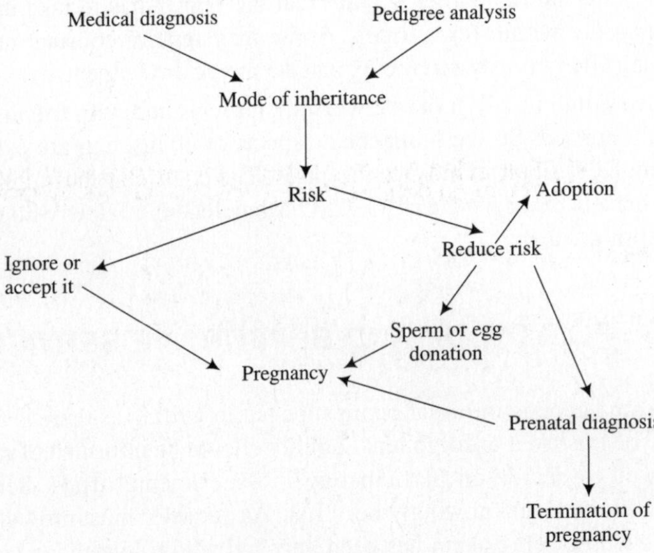


**Fig. 19.1** An overview of genetic counseling

CHAPTER 20

# Prenatal Diagnosis

## INTRODUCTION

The term 'prenatal diagnosis' refers to the ability to detect all genetic disorders before birth of the child. Prenatal diagnosis employs a variety of techniques to determine the health and condition of an unborn fetus. The ability to detect all major chromosomal anomalies and gene controlled biochemical defects has been a tremendous aid to genetic counseling. Such information can guide the family in reproductive decision making which may involve terminating the pregnancy, or facilitate planning of appropriate medical, surgical or psychological support.

Most pregnant women aged over 35 year are offered a scanning at about 18-20 weeks. If termination of pregnancy is advised then it is carried out as per "Pregnancy Termination Act" and beyond the 5 months period it is not safe for the carrying mother.

There are a variety of techniques available for prenatal diagnosis. Each of them can be applied only during specific time periods during the pregnancy for greatest utility.

In general they are classified as:

(i) Non-invasive techniques, those that do not require an incision or surgery

(ii) Invasive techniques often require incision or surgery.

## 20.1 NON-INVASIVE TECHNIQUES

### a. Radiography

When X-rays are used for detection, the technique is called radiography. This is often applied to detect skeletal deformities in the fetus. This technique can be adopted in two different ways.

### *i. Amniography*

Here a water soluble dye is introduced into the amnion. This material is swallowed by the fetus and the gastrointestinal tract can be visualized. This helps to diagnose gastrointestinal defects.

### *ii. Fetography*

This employs an oil soluble contrast material which adheres to the fetus and the outline of the fetus is viewed. It is useful in the recognition of limb abnormalities and other major malformations.

## b. Ultrasonography

This is useful in determining

(a) whether the fetus is alive
(b) fetal head size
(c) multiple births
(d) fetus position
(e) gross structural deformities
(f) amniotic fluid volume.

In ultrasound scanning sound waves of very high frequency for example several million cycles per second is applied. Echoes are reflected from organ boundaries and the degree of reflection depends on the thickness of the tissues. These are electronically transformed into an image in the computer monitor and a sonogram (scan) is developed. This technique is an integral part of all invasive techniques also.

Several anomalies like microcephaly, anencephaly, hydrocephaly, cleft lip, abnormalities of the brain, abdominal organs and heart are usually detectable.

There are some limitations to this technique. Some abnormalities without morphological manifestations like Down syndrome cannot be detected by ultrasonography.

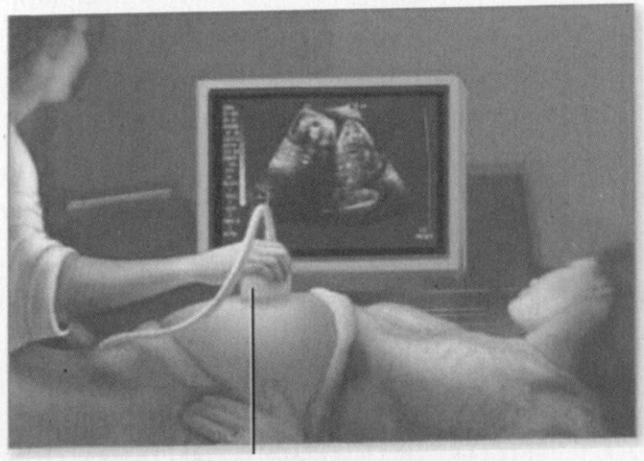


**Fig. 20.1** Ultrasound in pregnancy
(Source: www.nlm.nih.com)

### c. Screening of Maternal Blood

#### *i. AFP Test*

Maternal blood can provide useful indications. Alpha-fetoprotein is a protein produced by the fetal liver and can be traced in the maternal blood. If abnormally high level of AFP is detected then it indicates the occurrence of neural tube defects (NTD) in the fetus. The common NTD are

(1) Anencephaly - failure of the development of anterior part of brain

(2) Hydrocephaly - there is a heavy accumulation of cerebrospinal fluid in the head region

(3) Spina bifida - is the abnormal development of the lower part of the Spinal cord.

Measuring the level of AFP in the mother's blood would detect about 85% of these defects. Studies indicate that women who take folic acid on regular basis in early pregnancy may reduce this risk by 50%

#### *ii. Triple test*

This is a test where the level of three substances namely

(1) AFP

(2) HCG (human chorionic gonadotropin

(3) UE3 (unconjugated Estriol)

can be determined at 15$^{th}$ week of pregnancy. If an extra chromosome is present in the fetus as in the case of Down syndrome then the AFP level is low, HCG level is high and Estriol level tends to be lower. Triple test are valuable because 60 to 65 % pregnancies with Down syndrome can be detected.

#### *iii. Quadruple screen test*

Apart from measuring AFP, HCG and UE3, another substance namely Inhibin A can be measured in maternal serum. An increased level of Inhibin-A indicates trisomy-21.

**Table 20.1** The relationship between fetal condition and the level of the substances in maternal serum

| *Condition* | *AFP* | *UES* | *HCG* |
|---|---|---|---|
| Neural tube defect | Increased | Normal | Normal |
| Trisomy 21 | Low | Low | Increased |
| Trisomy 18 | Low | Low | Low |
| Molar pregnancy | Low | Low | Very high |
| Multiple gestation | Increased | Normal | Increased |
| Fetal death (stillbirth) | Increased | Low | Low |

## 20.2 INVASIVE TECHNIQUES

The accepted guidelines for invasive testing is that there must be some indications exist as in the following list before going for such procedures.

1. Maternal age is above 35 years at term.
2. Previous child with some chromosomal anomaly.
3. Family history of detectable genetic defect.
4. Family history of an X-linked disorder.
5. Elevated serum AFP or family history of NTD.
6. Consanguineous marriage.
7. Maternal illness or medication during pregnancy.
8. Abnormal amniotic fluid volume.

The following are the common invasive procedures:

## a. Amniocentesis

In recent years the availability of medical procedures such as amniocentesis has increased the effectiveness of counseling. The amniotic fluid that surrounds the fetus is about 200ml. It consists of fetal cells derived from the skin, respiratory and the urinary systems of the fetus. To obtain the cells, a long, thin needle is inserted through the pregnant woman's abdominal wall, uterus and fetal membranes by a medical practitioner and about 20ml of the amniotic fluid is withdrawn. The position of the fetus is monitored in the video screen by ultrasound scan. This is done often at 14$^{th}$ to 16$^{th}$ week of pregnancy. Cells from the sample are then grown in tissue culture and subsequently analyzed. Also, the fluid may be subjected to various biochemical tests.

In general the following tests are done:

1. Biochemical tests to detect enzyme or protein deficiency in inborn errors of metabolism like PKU and cysticfibrosis
2. Cells are processed for karyotyping and chromosome analysis is done for chromosomal disorders.
3. DNA analysis is performed to find out the gene mutation and carrier detection.
4. Fetal DNA is subjected to RFLP. For example in Beta thalassemia HpaI enzyme produces a 13kb long fragment in the Beta globin gene while in a normal person only 7.6 kb fragment is produced.
5. FISH uses Fluorescent labeled probes and the defective gene is identified by DNA hybridization.
6. The fluid may be subjected to AFP test.

These procedures may take about 3 weeks and just sufficient time is available for the couples to decide about therapeutic abortion.

This procedure is safe in a trained hand. Most women do not report the amniocentesis procedure to be painful. It usually takes a minute or less to perform. The risk for miscarriage from an amniocentesis is approximately 1 in 400 (0.25%). In the US approximately 30,000 women undergo amniocentesis.

## b. Chorionic Villus Sampling (CVS)

This procedure was first adopted in China in 1975 as a means of determining sex of a fetus. It is a specialized alternative test to amniocentesis. Here a biopsy is obtained from the placental tissue or like amniocentesis a needle is introduced and a bit of fetal tissue from the chorionic villi is sucked off from the placenta. The chorion is the fetal membrane with finger like projections namely the **chorionic villi** on the outerside. Both these are guided by ultrasound sonography. This is done in 9$^{th}$ to 12$^{th}$ week of pregnancy. The sample tissue is subjected to the tests as it is done in amniocentesis.

It is more advantageous than amniocentesis in that:

(i) It is performed in the early period of pregnancy.

(ii) It contains only fetal tissue.

(iii) The cells are actively dividing so chromosome study can be done without cell culture.

(iv) The results of the analysis are available much earlier for decision.

The CVS procedure takes a minute or two to perform and most women do not consider it to be painful. The risk of miscarriage out of CVS is 1 in 200 (0.5%).

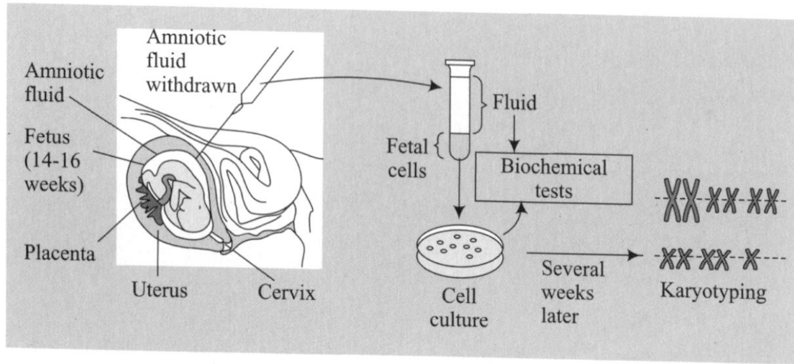


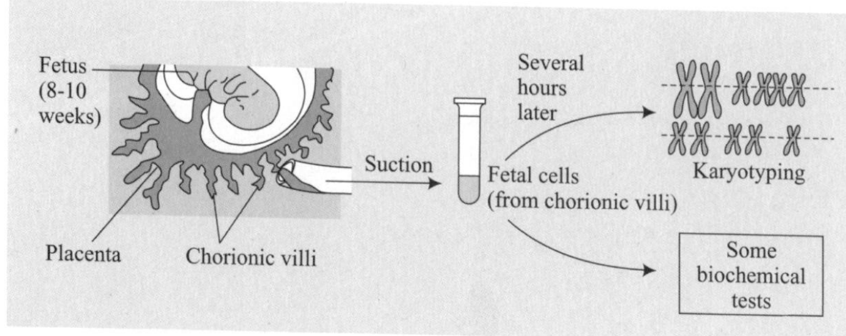


**Fig. 20.2** Amniocentesis (upper image) and chorionic villus sampling (lower image) (Source: www.anslem.edu)

## c. Fetoscopy

This is direct visualization of the external features of the fetus with the aid of a fine instrument the endoscope, introduced in to the amniotic sac. This is also used to obtain fetal blood samples, skin biopsies etc. The optimum age is 18-20 weeks of pregnancy and it carries a risk of 3% fetal loss.

## d. Preimplantation Genetic Diagnosis

In the context of 'test tube baby' (in vitro fertilization), one or two cells are collected when the embryo is 6-10 cells stage for direct examination by FISH, enabling selection of healthy embryos for implantation.

Flouresence in situ hybridization (FISH) is an advanced technique. The DNA sample of the fetus is obtained by the above mentioned procedures. Certain DNA probe prepared with flouresence can light up the corresponding DNA in the chromosome of the fetal cells. For example suppose if there are 3 'X' chromosomes in the fetus then there will be 3 bright spots or illuminated spots visualized in the microscope.

## e. Cordocentesis

From week 18 onwards a fetus sample can be taken by inserting fine needle transabdominally into the umbilical cord. This is carried with guidance by fetoscopy or ultrasonography. There is 3% risk of miscarriage. Culture of extracted cells for few days provides material suitable for chromosomal studies or DNA analysis.

CHAPTER 21

# Management of Genetic Diseases

## INTRODUCTION

In principle, genetically influenced conditions can be treated. Effective therapy usually requires an understanding of causes and effects. With all the advancement in molecular genetics only 12% of the genetic diseases could be considered for treatment. Those that responded partially to treatment increased from 40% to 57% over the decade. The success rate is very low. Some of the better known genetic diseases, like Down syndrome, Muscular dystrophy etc. remain untreatable. It would be best if genetic diseases could be prevented from occurring. Prevention becomes a matter of genetic testing and counseling. These may include prenatal diagnosis, selective abortion and alternative reproductive technologies.

**Table 21.1** List of the available means of treatment for the genetic diseases

| *Means of treatment* | *Disease* |
|---|---|
| 1. Surgical therapy | |
| (i) Surgical repair | Cleft lip and cleft palate |
| (ii) Removal of spleen | Spherocytosis |
| (iii) Removal of colon | Familial polyposis |
| 2. Drug therapy | |
| (i) Hydroxy urea | Sickle cell disease |
| (ii) Beta blockers | Hypertension |

*(Contd.)*

*(Contd.)*

| | |
|---|---|
| 3. Dietary restriction | |
| (i) Phenylalanine | Phenylketonuria |
| (ii) Fava beans | G6PD deficiency |
| 4. Depletion of an excessive substance | |
| (i) Copper | Wilson disease |
| (ii) Uric acid | Gout |
| 5. Replacement of a missing gene product | |
| (i) Insulin | Diabetes |
| (ii) Clotting factor viii | Hemophilia |
| 6. Organ and tissue transplantation | |
| (i) Bone marrow | Beta thalassemia |
| | SCID |
| (ii) Liver | Alpha-1- antitrypsin deficiency |
| 7. Antisense therapy | Crohn disease |
| 8. Gene therapy | ADA deficiency |

## 21.1 THERAPEUTIC MEASURES

### i. Surgical Therapy

The disfiguring due to a defect may be corrected by surgery. The disfigurement, speech difficulties and swallowing problems of cleft lip and cleft palate can be restored by skillful surgery. The extra digits of polydactyly can be easily removed. In the autosomal dominant disorder spherocytosis, the RBC become fragile and often leads to chronic anemia and gallstones at an early age. Removal of the spleen allows the red blood cells to survive longer and relieves most of the disease symptoms.

a. Baby with cleft lip

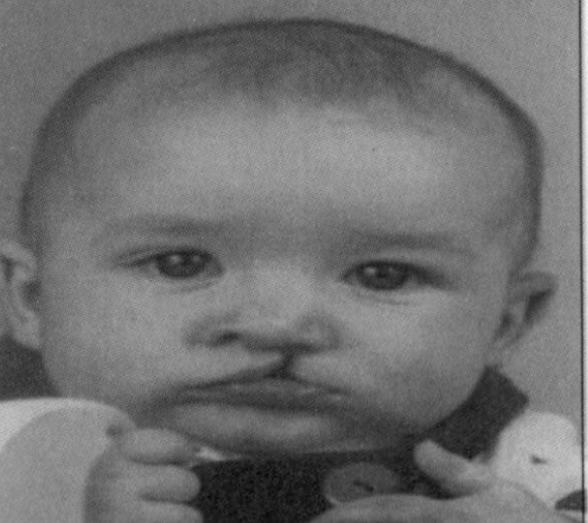

b. After surgical therapy

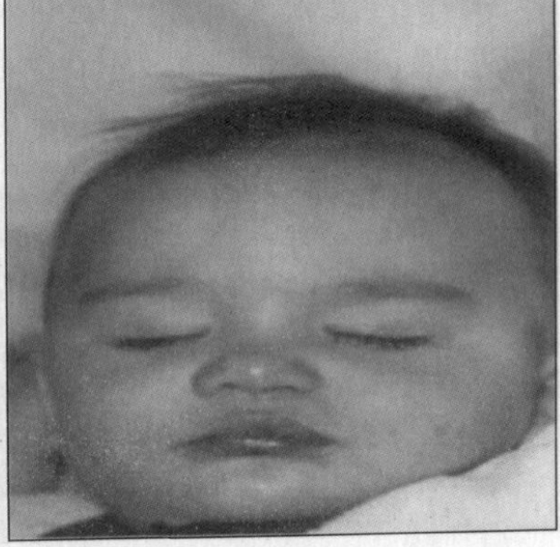

**Fig. 21.1** Surgical therapy for cleft lip
(Source: www.revolution.health.com)

## ii. Drug Therapy

Some genetic diseases can be managed by drugs. In hypertension, beta blockers can be used to reduce the activity of the heart and thereby reduce the pressure on the aorta.

Hydroxyurea is used in treatment of sickle-cell disease. This drug increases the production of fetal haemoglobin, thus reducing the sickling of red blood cells caused by abnormal beta globin chains.

## iii. Dietary Restriction

The diet therapy for PKU is an example for this type of treatment. In patients with PKU, an enzyme deficiency reduces the conversion of phenylalanine to tyrosine, so that phenylalanine accumulates to a toxic level. The low-phenylalanine diet prevents this accumulation. The recommended diet lowers drastically the intake of the amino acid phenylalanine which is a component of proteins.

## iv. Depletion of Excessive Substance

Wilson's disease, a rare recessive genetic disorder is due to an error in copper metabolism. In affected persons, the abnormal deposition of copper causes liver and brain damage, if untreated it leads to death. A drug namely pencillamine when given, binds to copper and lead to its excretion in the urine. Early diagnosis and treatment can prevent the serious consequences of Wilson's disease

Heterozygotes for hypercholesterolemia have accumulation of cholesterol to a high level. This leads to atherosclerosis that is hardening of blood vessels and may result in heart attacks beginning in 30 years of age. The symptoms are due to excessive LDL (low density lipoprotein). Number of drugs are available in the market when used, reduces the serum cholesterol level.

## v. Replacement of a Missing Gene Product

In Diabetes the missing gene product is insulin. Recombinant DNA techniques have been used to make insulin and injection of this insulin to a diabetic will supply the missed insulin.

Similarly in Hemophilia A the missing blood clotting factor viii (antihemophilic globulin) could be supplied. Though an expensive therapy, biotechnologically produced clotting factor viii is available for treatment.

A novel method of delivery of the therapeutic agent has been used in the treatment of ADA deficiency. The normal ADA (adenosine deaminase) enzyme is involved in the purine metabolism, and its deficiency affects the production of T cells and B cells. As a result, ADA deficient children succumb to viral, bacterial and fungal infections. Their immune system becomes deficient due to impaired antibody production. To treat this disease ADA enzyme isolated from cow is injected regularly. The enzyme is first coated with polyethelene glycol (PEG) so that the life time of the enzyme is prolonged.

## vi. Organ and Tissue Transplantation

An interesting medical procedure for transferring the correct genetic information into patients who have a hereditary disease is to transplant an organ or tissue from a normal individual. Such a graft may provide a missing enzyme or protein within the patient's body on a continuing basis.

For example a 'bubble boy' with **Severe Combined Immunodeficiency (SCID) disease** could receive a bone marrow from his sister or brother. In SCID the functioning of B cells and T cells is impaired and so the child is prone to all infections. The bone marrow when transplanted will supply functional B cells and T cells.

Bone marrow transplant is also attempted to treat thalassemia.

**Alpha- 1- antitrypsin defeciency** causes a thick secretion of mucus in the respiratory tract and results in cystic fibrosis symptoms. This enzyme is produced in the liver. So a liver transplant is the treatment method for this disease.

### vii. Antisense Therapy

This is formulated in 1980s. In protein synthesis, mRNA carries the essential information to carry out translation in the process of protein production. Synthesis of a harmful protein (responsible for the disease) can be blocked by short nucleotide segments of about 20 base called oligonucleotides that are complementary to a portion of the mRNA. Complementarity leads to binding, which invites a normal cell enzyme, to break down the mRNA. Because the mRNA is often called the sense molecule, the treatment approach is called **antisense therapy**.

Clinical trials of antisense therapy for **Crohn disease** have been successful. This disorder results in chronic inflammation of the bowel, leading to abdominal pain, diarrohea, fever and general weakness. It affects the intestine mostly. The antisense treatment attacks the mRNA that encodes a cell adhesion protein involved in the inflammatory process.

Antisense therapy is being investigated for a wide variety of genetic and non-genetic diseases, including cancers, cardiovascular conditions, thalassemia and AIDS.

### viii. Gene Therapy

This is a cure for genetic diseases. A normal gene is supplied which will produce normal protein to do the normal function. Somatic gene therapy is done using body cells to carry the correct gene. The same methodology can be adopted to germ cells then called germinal gene therapy.

Gene therapy has been successfully performed for ADA deficiency. The first human trail of gene therapy was begun in 1990. A Four year old girl was given gene therapy. ADA is adenosine deaminase enzyme necessary for the functioning of T cells. The T cells are involved in immunological response to fight against an infection. The deficiency of this enzyme causes immunodeficiency. The treatment procedure involves in vitro technique.

The following steps are involved in Gene therapy:

1. Isolation of T cells from the blood of a patient.
2. Then these cells are cultured in the laboratory.
3. Simultaneously a vector is prepared by genetic manipulation.

   The widely used vector is a retrovirus and is genetically modified. The gene for ADA is artificially synthesized and introduced into the retrovirus genome which becomes the carrier of this gene.
4. This retrovirus usually MMLV (Moloney Murine Leukemia Virus) is allowed to infect the T cells in the culture. Many retroviruses infect target cells with nearly 100% efficiency. The T cells carrying the ADA gene from the retrovirus is the gene corrected cells.

5. These cells are then returned to the patient by blood transfusion.

This treatment requires repeated injection of gene corrected T cells. To overcome this problem bone marrow stem cells from which these T lymphocytes are derived are subjected to gene therapy instead of just T cells.

Hundreds of protocols for gene therapy involving thousands of patients worldwide are now in progress. For cystic fibrosis trials, the vector is an adenovirus (cold virus) carrying the corrected CFTR gene that is sprayed directly into the patient's airway (in vivo technique). An advantage of adenovirus is that they infect non-dividing lung cells (which retrovirus does not). However the adenovirus does not persist in infected cells, so that the therapeutic treatment must be repeated often and may cause serious immunological reactions and infections.

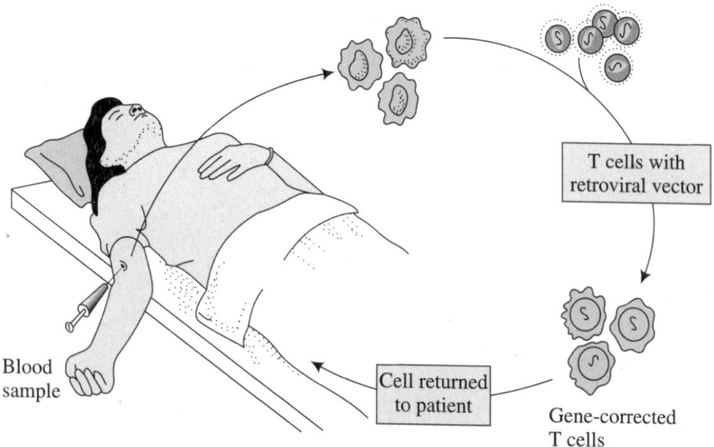


**Fig. 21.2** Gene therapy protocol
(Adapted from Mangae, E.J. and A.P. Mangae, 1999)

**Table 21.2** Human gene therapy trials

| *Disease* | *Gene therapy* |
|---|---|
| Severe combined immunodeficiency (SCID) | Adenosine deaminase (ADA) |
| Cystic fibrosis | Cystic fibrosis transmembrane regulator (CFTR) |
| Familial hypercholesterolemia | Low density lipoprotein (LDL) receptor |
| Emphysema | alpha-1-antitrypsin |
| Hemophilia B | Clotting Factor IX |
| Thalassemia | alpha and beta globin |
| Sickle cell anemia | beta globin |
| Melanoma | Tumor necrosis factor (TNF) |
| Duschenne muscular dystrophy | Dystrophin |
| Lesch Nyhan syndrome | HGPRT enzyme |

CHAPTER 22

# Ethical Aspects in Genetic Counseling

## INTRODUCTION

Presently, genetic counseling goes beyond mere presentations of risk facts and figures to the prevention and cure of disease, the relief of pain and the maintenance of health. For many disorders it is only possible to give precise recurrence risk conditions and also the order of risk, if extensive family studies are available. Moral, Ethical and Philosophical aspects involved in genetic counseling are now emerging as major issues with the development of the application of various diagnostic techniques as amniocentesis and CVS during pregnancy. The consultee and the counselor are now faced with choices that were once left to fate. Should the genetically defective be aborted? Do parents have a right to produce defective children?

## 22.1 ETHICS IN PRENATAL DIAGNOSIS

When genetic risks are high, the desire to have a healthy child and avoid danger of oneself, family and society are frequently in conflict. Although 96% of the counseling sessions end well with no very little chances for the occurrence of the disease, the remaining 4% people in the high risk category are left with three options: (i) prenatal diagnosis and abortion if required, (ii) artificial insemination and (iii) gene therapy

### Prenatal Diagnosis (PND) and Abortion Choices

The choice to abort any pregnancy is a moral problem wherever duties to protect the interests of the woman, the fetus and the society are held to be in conflict. Historically some of the earliest conflicts about PND were on the question of whether abortion was its primary goal. One group argued that the destruction of certain fetuses was the morally unacceptable goal of PND outweighing the possibility that it might give reassurance to some at-risk parents that their child would (likely) be unaffected. The other group contended that since PND was done largely with an intention to abort an affected fetus, the practice contradicted the basic purpose of medicinal science.

With the involvement of euthenics, i.e. state-of-the-art of treatment for genetic disorders by modification of the environment to allow the genetically abnormal individual to develop normally and to live a relatively normal life, abortion choices will become predictably more complicated. Euthenics can be applied both medically and socially and examples of phenylketouria (PKU) treatment by diet control, use of human growth hormone for growth disorders, purified factor viii for haemophilia A, etc., illustrate medical euthenics, while special schools for deaf children, illustrate social euthenics.

Access of PND and genetic service is the central moral problem in medical ethics. Except for Denmark where about 80% of the women who need PND receive it, most of the countries do not meet the true need for services. Further, women who undergo PND belong largely to higher economic groups. Lack of financial resources and adequate planning have restricted the distribution of genetic services in almost every country.

Research in the context of clinical trials raises ethical issues. A randomized clinical trial requires careful consideration because a proven new approach will be withheld by chance, from some in order to compare its advantages and disadvantages. Clinical research in prenatal care presents special complexities because the fetus as well as the pregnant woman are the subject of research.

## 22.2 PROBLEMS FACED BY THE COUNSELOR

There cannot be a universal model for genetic counseling because counseling is an understanding of a set of facts according to the counselor's frame of reference, background in the science of genetics, and previous training and experience in effectively communicating with the consultee. In order to communicate effectively, the counselor must consider the educational background of the consultee, what to disclose and how to limit the ways in which he can communicate. It has been found that the principle obstacles to the effective use of genetic counseling are emotional conflicts, and lack of knowledge of genetics and biology.

An equally difficult assignment for the counselor is presenting his knowledge in an unbiased manner. It is difficult for a counselor to impart unbiased information because of the consultee's personal and family history such as parental age, ethnic background, reproductive history, i.e. abortions, stillborn or dead siblings, and the age, sex and health of the living children. This may lead the counselor to adopt a directive rather than a non-directive approach to genetic counseling. The major difference between directive and non-directive counseling is whether or not the counselor actively participates or helps the consultees to make a decision. Directive counseling has a positive influence on the consultee's decision. The non-directive approach involves presentation of the facts in an unbiased manner, leaving the entire responsibility of decision with the consultee. During counseling, the counselor may come across other findings that may put him in a situation of ethical dilemma. Some of these are fetal sex, findings of questionable or potentially harmful significance, false paternity, etc.

Is there a duty to disclose fetal sex to parents, since this finding is not related to any disease, except in x-linked disorders? Should physicians cooperate with the desire of the parents to know the fetal sex, especially when they have reason to suspect that some parents will misinterpret the indication and seek abortion elsewhere for undesired gender?

Another difficult conflict involves ambiguous sex. Should they be told? Will a full biological explanation harm their self-esteem and damage them psychologically?

Medical geneticists learn many family secrets, such as previous abortions, previous abnormal births and occasional false paternity. The findings can be made after PND of a recessive disorder and testing the carrier parents or in the context of genetic screening after the birth of an affected infant. The putative father believes that he must be a carrier, but tests are negative. The option left is partial or total deception. Should the family be protected from the disruption due to disclosure, with the risk of inappropriate decisions about future child bearing being based on false information?

## 22.3 GUIDANCE IN GENETIC COUNSELING

A proposal for guidelines for PND, genetic counseling and screening has been made. The proposal assumes that consensus exists among medical geneticists, obstetricians and parents about some key ethical principles and approaches to difficult choices: (1) Parental autonomy in abortion choices; (2) Non-directive counseling; (3) PND that must be provided when parents need the information to prepare themselves for the birth of a possibly affected child; (4) Practitioners need to disclose to the consultee the risk and benefits of each procedure in PND; (5) information of xy females and xx males with great care that casts no ambiguity on the patient's social and phenotypic sexual identity; (6) In case putative father is not the biological father of the fetus the mother to be informed first to avoid social problems and she may be left to take final decision; (7) Medical geneticists to decide which of the disorders warrants the options of prenatal diagnosis and termination of pregnancy, and (8) Consequences from the above to be evaluated in terms of basic ethical principles, and critical tests of what is best for the individuals, groups and society.

### Conclusions

Application of science and scientific principle has two faces. To decide the correct use, man must deal with his conscious, individual and social status and the ethics underlying the applications.

Genetic counseling is a practical method of calculating risk figures, intended for information regarding the unborn, and we ought to use it in an efficient manner but in a direction, which our ethics and morality point to. The decision taken by the parents after the counseling session must leave them satisfied instead of placing them in a state of dilemma.

CHAPTER 23

# Assisted Reproductive Technology

## INTRODUCTION

One of the greatest advances in reproductive medicine is Assisted Reproductive Technology (ART). Due to immense advances in the field of infertility, the impossible has been made possible. The pioneer in this field is Dr. Patrick Christopher Steptoe (1913-1988) who programmed the world's first test tube baby by In vitro Fertilization. The world's first test tube baby Louise Brown was born in London in July 1978. At present thousands of test tube babies are born from frozen embryos.

## 23.1 FERTILITY

Pregnancy results from the union of sperm and ovum (egg). In the female ovum is produced every month due to hormonal changes. Eggs are contained within little sacs, called follicles, deep in the ovaries. Each month one follicle dominates and starts to grow, ruptures and releases the egg. This cyclic event is under the control of two pituitary hormones namely Follicle stimulating hormone (FSH) and Leutinizing hormone (LH). These hormones in turn stimulate the ovaries to produce two other hormones Oestrogen and Progesterone. These hormones bring about the monthly growth and shedding of the endometrium, the inner layer of the uterus.

The ovum is released from the ovary and is picked up by the mobile, finger-like processes called fimbriae at the end of the fallopian tubes. If intercourse has taken place, the sperm in the vagina will swim up through the uterus into the fallopian tubes and fertilize the egg at the fimbrial end.

The fertilized egg then travels slowly down the fallopian tube towards the uterus assisted by the small hair-like processes called cilia within the tubes. This process takes about 4-5 days. The fertilized egg reaches the uterus and gets buried itself into the prepared layer of the uterus, and grow into a baby. This process is called implantation. If fertilization and implantation do not occur then the menstrual flow starts.

## 23.2 INFERTILITY

Infertility is the inability to conceive a child.

### a. Male Infertility

Infertility in the male is easy to detect but harder to treat than female infertility.

1. **Oligospermia**: This is reduced concentration of sperms in the semen. A fertile man produces a semen sample that has 1-3 ml, 60 to 120 million sperms/ml, sperm motility is 80% and abnormal sperm is below 40%.
2. **Azospermia**: Sperm quality is even more important than quantity. Sperm cells that are unable to move can not reach the ovum.
3. Male infertility is also due to a varicose vein in the scrotum. This enlarged vein brings too much heat to developing sperm and they can not mature.
4. Sometimes a man's immune system produces antibodies that cover the sperm and prevent them binding to ovum.

### b. Female Infertility

Female infertility can be due to abnormalities in any part of the reproductive system.

1. **Irregular ovulation**: This is due to hormonal imbalance. This is caused by a tumor in the ovary or in the pituitary gland or underactive thyroid gland or steroid based drugs. Sometimes a woman produces prolactin, the hormone that normally promotes milk production and suppresses ovulation.
2. **Abnormal fallopian tube**: The common problem is tubal block. Fallopian tube may be blocked due to birth defect or, more likely by infection. In this case the sperm and ovum can not meet or the fertilized ovum can not descend to the uterus and results in ectopic pregnancy.
3. **Problems in uterus**: Implantation of the fertilized egg is not possible if the uterus lining is not normal. Excess tissue growth is caused by benign tumors, called fibroids or endometriosis where tissue builds up in the uterus.

4. **Cervical problems**: The cervix is the narrow outlet at the lower end of the uterus through which the sperm has to pass. The cervix produces thick mucus which prevents the sperm movement. Sometimes vaginal secretions are acidic or alkaline that sperms are weakened or killed.
5. **Antisperm antibody (ASAB)**: ASAB is produced against the sperms in the women's body. ASAB immobilizes the sperms.

## 23.3 REPRODUCTIVE TECHNOLOGIES

The treatment of infertility is fast growing field in reproductive medicine and numerous methods are available to treat any kind of infertility. The techniques involved are termed **Assisted Reproductive Technology (ART).**

### i. Intrauterine Insemination (IUI)

This is the oldest alternate method of reproduction. A woman who desires to have a child and whose partner is infertile receives the sperm from an anonymous donor. The first artificial insemination in humans was done in 1890. Today donated sperm is frozen and stored in sperm banks which provide sperms for insemination. A couple who prefers artificial insemination can select sperm from a catalog that gives the characteristics of donors.

The women are usually superovulated by administering gonodotropins. This causes multiple egg development. The semen is washed and the highly motile sperms are selected. With the help of a thin catheter, the sperms are placed either in the cervix or in the uterine cavity.

### ii. Surrogate Motherhood

A surrogate mother helps when a woman's uterus fails to maintain pregnancy while the male partner produces healthy sperms. A surrogate mother is artificially inseminated with sperm donated by the man. When the child is born, the surrogate gives the baby to the couple. The surrogate is both genetic and gestational mother.

Alternately a surrogate mother lends only her uterus, receiving a fertilized egg conceived from a man and a woman who has healthy ovaries but lacks a functional uterus. Here the surrogate mother is only a gestational mother and returns the baby to the donors.

### iii. *In Vitro* Fertilization (IVF) and Embryo Transfer (ET)

In IVF, The egg from woman is removed, fertilized in the laboratory, and then the fertilized egg is returned to the uterus. IVF means 'fertilization in glass'. A woman undergoes IVF if the ovaries and uterus work but the fallopian tubes are blocked.

To perform IVF more eggs are required. To achieve this, the ovaries are hyperstimulated by injecting hormones. The hormones induce superovulation. The following drug regime is adopted to induce superovulation. Clomiphene citrate, Human menopausal gonadotropin, Follicle stimulating hormone and Gonadotropin releasing agonists are used to induce ovulation. Using a laparoscope, a physician removes several of the oocytes and transfers them to a laboratory dish. Chemicals that mimic the female reproductive tract are added, and sperm donated are applied to the oocytes. The successful fertilization is indicated by the presence of two pronuclei within the developing embryo.

The embryos in 8 cell stage are transferred to the uterus between 48-60 hours following insemination. The transfer procedure is carried out by the use of a catheter. Generally not more than three embryos are transferred.

The success rate of IVF is about 15-20%. The low success rate is due to the following reasons namely increased risk of abortion, multiple pregnancy, ectopic pregnancy, low birth weight baby and premature delivery.

By employing IVF and ET, the world's first test tube baby, Louise Brown was born in UK on 28th July 1978. The world's second test tube baby, Durga was born in Kolkata on 3rd October 1978.

IVF is one of the major achievements of medical sciences in the last century. It has become a novel way of treating infertility. Today, there are more than million test tube babies born all over the world.

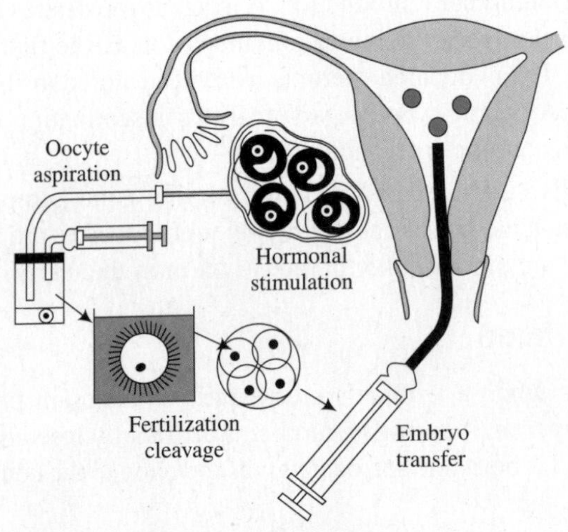


**Fig. 23.1** In vitro fertilization and embryo transfer (Source: www.ivf.net.com)

## iv. Gamete Intrafallopian Transfer (GIFT)

In the mid-1980s, Richardo Asch, at the University of Texas, developed a procedure called GIFT, which stands for gamete intrafallopian transfer. In GIFT fertilization is assisted, but it occurs in the woman's body rather than in glassware. GIFT involves the transfer of both sperm and unfertilized egg into the fallopian tube. This allows the fertilization to naturally occur *in vivo*. The prerequisite for GIFT is that the woman should have at least one normal fallopian tube.

In GIFT, superovulation drugs are given to a woman for a week and then several of the eggs are removed. From a sperm donor, most active sperms are separated. The collected eggs and sperms are deposited together in the woman's fallopian tube. GIFT is about 40% successful and half the cost of IVF.

### v. Zygote Intrafallopian Transfer (ZIFT)

A variation of GIFT is ZIFT. Here an *in vitro* fertilized ovum is introduced into the woman's fallopian tube. ZIFT is suitable when the infertility lies in men or in case of failure of GIFT. The woman's eggs are exposed to her husband's sperms in the laboratory. The fertilized eggs within 24 hours are transferred to the fallopian tube by laparoscopy.

### vi. Intravaginal Culture (IVC)

In IVC the body's own environment is appropriately utilized. The collected eggs and sperms are placed in a culture medium inside a sealed container. This is inserted into the vagina and is held by a vaginal diaphragm. The sperms and ova are maintained at the normal body temperature in contrast to the laboratory condition. After three days the container is opened, and the fertilized and dividing zygotes are transferred into the uterus.

### vii. Cytoplasmic Transfer (CT)

The cytoplasm of a cell includes vital organelles. Mitochondria is one if the organelles which provides energy to the cell. The deficiency in the mitochondria may result in the impairment of cell division of zygote after fertilization. This may result in abnormal cell division and poor development of embryo. In CT, the cytoplasm with active mitochondria from a donor is transferred into the ovum of a woman. The advantage is that the mother's own genetic material is passed on to the offspring.

The CT is achieved either by transferring a small amount of cytoplasm by a tiny needle from a donor to a recipient oocyte or by applying electricity a large amount of cytoplasm from a donor is fused with the recipient's cytoplasm.

### viii. Intracytoplasmic Sperm Injection (ICSI)

ICSI is a novel technology in treating infertility. ICSI is preferred over other techniques to treat male infertility. In this procedure the zona pellucida (outer layer of the ovum) is opened using either chemicals or a sharp instrument. This is called partial zona dissection (PZD). A single spermatozoon can be directly injected into the cytoplasm of the ovum through the micropuncture of the zona pellucida. A micropipette is used to hold the egg in position while the sperm is injected into the cytoplasm.

ICSI is the most successful technique with 65% success rate. ICSI has revolutionized ART by utilizing the sperms of men who were once considered to be unsuitable for fertilization.

### ix. Subzonal Inaertion (SUZI)

In SUZI, the zona pellucida is punctured and sperms about 1-30 in number are injected into area between the zona and the egg.

### x. Round Spermid Nucleus Injection (ROSNI)

Some persons have zero sperm count. For these men, it is possible to take out the round spermatids which are immature sperms, directly from the testicle. The nucleus from the spermatid is isolated that contains the genetic material and is injected into the egg. ROSNI is a recent achievement in the treatment of male infertility through micromanipulation.

### xi. Micromanipulation

This technique involves *in vitro* microsurgically assisted fertilization procedures. This is required when the sperms are unable to penetrate the zona pellucida of oocyte and fertilize. Micromanipulation is adopted in sever cases of male infertility.

### xii. Cryopreservation

Preserving tissues in a frozen state is termed cryopreservation. This is very useful in ART. Before the commencement of treatment, the semen or eggs from a donor, fertilized eggs could be collected and cryopreserved. Embryos can also be preserved for transfer at a later stage. Human embryos have been successfully cryopreserved. In cryopreservation chemicals called as **cryoprotectants** such as 1, 2-propanediol or dimethyl sulfoxide or glycerol are used. They are stored in -196°C under liquid nitrogen. At appropriate time the sperm or egg or embryos are retrieved, thawed, cryoprotectants washed off and then transferred. Many test tube babies have been born as a result of this freezing technology.

### xiii. Assisted Hatching (AH)

One of the problems in the success of ART is improper implantation of the embryos in the uterus. AH is a novel technique for the proper implantation of the embryo in the uterus. The step necessary for implantation is the removal of zona pellucida. In certain women, especially above 40 years of age, natural hatching does not occur and requires assistance. AH is carried out by using LASER to make small hole in the zona pellucida. These embryos when transferred into the uterus, hatch and get implanted.

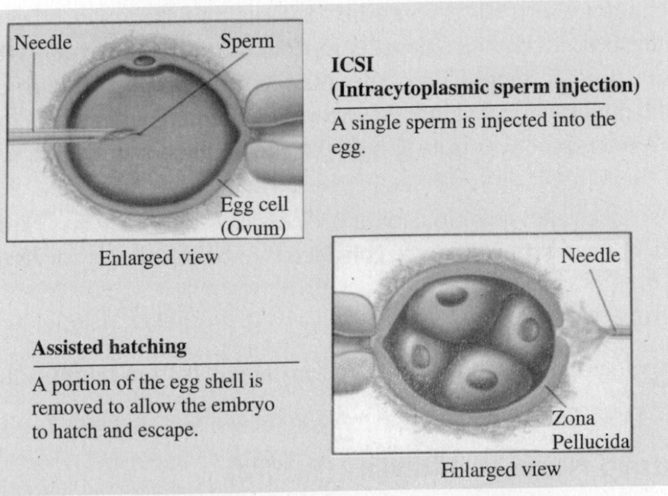


**Fig. 23.2** Intracytoplasmic sperm injection (ICSI) and assisted hatching (AH) (Source: www.auto-medical-rss.blogspot.com)

### xiv. Preimplantation Genetic Diagnosis (PGD)

Reproductive technologies make possible earlier detection of genetic and chromosomal abnormalities, even before the pre-embryo implants in the uterus on the sixth day. This new medical tool is called PGD. A direct determination of chromosomal anomalies prior to implantation ensures successful pregnancy and delivery of a healthy baby. In this technique, a cell from an 8-cell pre-embryo is removed and its DNA is amplified by Polymerase chain reaction and probed for genetic information without damaging the remaining 7cells. The pre-embryos which are free of genetic illness is implanted in the uterus and allowed to continue development. The first children who had PGD were born in 1990. PGD is useful in the diagnosis of several genetic diseases like cystic fibrosis, sickle cell anemia, hemophilia and Duchenne muscular dystrophy.

PGD is highly advantageous in genetic counseling, since the embryos with genetic disorders can be eliminated in the early stages of development without the formation of offsprings with undesirable characteristics.

## 23.4 LIMITATIONS OF ART

There are certain disadvantages associated with ART in humans. But the merits overweigh the demerits.

- Due to administration of hormones and drugs, ovarian hyperstimulation is frequently associated with complications and some times life threatening. This is called Ovarian hyperstimulation syndrome (OHSS).
- ART is also associated with multiple pregnancies, increased risk of anemia, gestational diabetes and premature labor. Low birth weight and prematurity is linked with mortality and morbidity.
- The use of fertility drugs and injuries to ovary increase the risk of ovarian cancer.
- Controlled ovarian stimulation (COH) causes multiple follicular utility. There is a risk of premature menopause as COH may reduce the ovarian follicles, besides speeding up aging.

CHAPTER 24

# Stem Cells

## INTRODUCTION

Stem cells science is a revolutionary science that has been developed over the past two years. This science is galloping at a high speed. Stem cells promise to be a powerful new technology. Stem cells are very promising in treating debilitating diseases like Alzheimer's disease, Cancer, Parkinson's disease. Type1 Diabetes, Spinalcord injury, Stroke, Burns, Heart disease, Osteoarthritis and Rheumatoid arthritis. Today, donated organs and tissues are often used to replace those that are diseased or destroyed. Unfortunately, the number of people needing transplants far exceeds the number of organs available. Stem cells offer the potential for supplying cells and tissues, which can be used to treat these various tissues.

## 24.1 HISTORY

The first embryonic stem cells from mammals were isolated from mice in 1981. It took another 14 years before embryonic stem cells were isolated from non-Human primates, with a breakthrough resulting from experimenting on the Rhesus monkey in 1995, followed by the Mormoset monkey in 1996. Using the same techniques with 14 human blastocysts produced by IVF programs resulted in the isolation of five human embryonic stem cell line in 1998. The study of human stem cells has just begun.

### What are Stem Cells?

Most of the 300 trillion cells of the body have 220 types and they have specialized functions. Blood, Lung, Brain, Skin, or Liver cells are specialized for what they do. They can not do anything other than what they were designed for. On the other hand, stem cells are undifferentiated "blank" cells that do not yet have a specific function. They are like a blank microchip that can ultimately be programmed to perform any number of specialized tasks. They are "all purpose" cells. Additionally, stem cells are self-sustaining and can replicate themselves for long periods of time.

## 24.2 TYPES

### a. Embryonic Stem Cells

All human beings start their lives from a single cell, called the zygote, which is formed after fertilization. The zygote divides repeatedly and about five days after conception, there is a hollow ball of about 150 cells and is called the blastocyst.This consists of a layer of trophoblast cells and the inner cell mass (ICM). Embryonic stem cells are the cells that make the inner cell mass. As embryonic stem cells they can form all cell types in an adult, they are referred to as pluripotent stem cells.

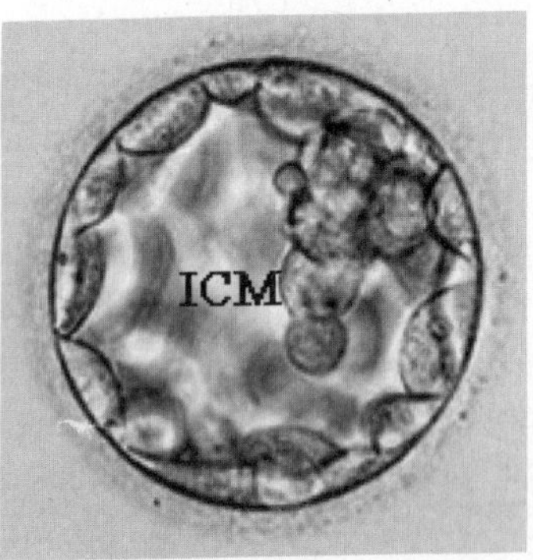


**Fig. 24.1** Blastocyst showing inner cell mass (Source: www.advancedfertility.com)

### b. Adult Stem Cells

Stem cells can be also found in very small numbers in various tissues in the adult body. For example, bone marrow stem cells are found in the marrow of the bone and they give rise to all specialized blood cell types. Adult stem cells are typically programmed to perform different cell types of their own tissue; they are called multipotent stem cells.

### c. Other Types

Stem cells can be also obtained from sources like umbilical cord of a new born baby. This is an accessible source of stem cells. Recently, scientists have discovered the existence of stem cells in baby teeth and in amniotic fluid.

## Stem Cell Bank

Human cord blood, neural stem cells and human embryonic stem cell banks have been established in various countries and are currently being expanded. Cord blood, like bone marrow, is stored as source of hematopoietic stem cells for the treatment of specific genetic and acquired diseases.

Cord blood banking is an alien concept till a few years ago in India is becoming popular. It is built around the possibility of use either by same child at a later date or by siblings who are either already sick or may require it in case they have genetic, hematologic or oncology disorders. Storing cord blood is a "biological insurance". Treating genetic or other diseases using cord blood may become a reality in future.

## Stem Cell Line

A stem cell line is composed of a population of stem cells that can replicate themselves for a long period of time *in vitro*. To date, over 100 human embryonic stem cell lines have been derived world wide. However only 22 cell lines are adequately characterized and are eligible for federal funding in USA. Detailed information on those 22 cell lines can be found at the National Institutes of Human Stem cell Registry, USA.

## Stem Cell Culture

Stem cells are grown in culture dishes in incubators at 37°c under high humidity. Since there are many different types of stem cells, the components of the culture medium for each type of stem cells are different.

Human embryonic stem cells can be grown as small colonies on layers of skin cells in the presence of serum. The skin cells are "feeder cells" which provide unknown growth factors and together with serum nourish the stem cells in their undifferentiated state. The cells are maintained by "passaging".

Haematopoietic stem cells can be derived from bone marrow, placenta or umbilical cord and cultured.

Human mesenchyme stem cells or bone marrow stem cells, are grown for several weeks and these cells attach to the plastic on the bottom of the culture dishes.

Human neural stem cells can be grown from fetal or adult brain tissue in culture media. They grow in suspension and they do not need serum. In culture, one single neural stem cell can divide to make more cells that together form a round hollow structure known as neurosphere. Neurospheres continue to grow in culture and when they get too big, are disaggregated into single cells. These single cells are mixed population of neural stem cells and mature cells. The neural stem cells can be selected from this mixed population and once again grown into rounded and hollow neurospheres. This process of disaggregation and neurosphere formation can be repeated several times. Eventually all the neural stem cells differentiate into more mature cells.

## 24.3 POTENTIAL USES OF HUMAN STEM CELLS

### a. Cell Therapy

Stem cells can be used to generate healthy and functioning specialized cells, which can replace diseased or dysfunctional cells. Replacing diseased cells with healthy cells, called **cell therapy**, is similar to the process of organ transplantation except that here, there is transplantation of cells. Stem cells can serve as an alternate renewable source for specialized cells. Currently, researchers are investigating the use of adult, fetal and embryonic stem cells as a source for various, specialized cell types, such as nerve cells, muscle cells, blood cells and skin cells that can be used to treat various diseases.

Advances in stem cell technologies have the potential to revolutionize medicine.

Some examples of treatments for major diseases from stem cell technologies are outlined below.

**Type I Diabetes:** Type I Diabetes is an autoimmune disease characterized by destruction of insulin producing cells in the pancreas. Current efforts to treat patients with pancreas transplants, which is limited by the small number of donated pancreas and the toxicity of immunosuppressive drug treatments required to prevent organ rejection. It is hoped that pluripotent stem cells, instructed to differentiate into a particular pancreatic cell called a beta cell, could overcome the shortage of material to transplant.

**Nervous system disease:** Many of these diseases result from the loss of nerve cells, as mature nerve cells can not divide to replace those that are lost. In Parkinson's disease, nerve cells that make the chemical dopamine die. In Alzheimer's disease, cells that are responsible for the production of certain neurotransmitters die. In spinal cord injury, brain trauma and even stroke, many different types of cells are lost to die. It is thought that perhaps the only hope for treating such individuals comes from the potential to create new nerve tissue restoring function from pluripotent stem cells.

**Primary immunodeficiency diseases:** There are more than 70 different forms of congenital and inherited deficiencies of the immune system that have been recognized, and are complicated to treat. These diseases are characterized by an unusual susceptibility to infection. However, the transplantation of stem cells reconstituted with the normal gene could result in restoration of life span and quality of life for these people.

**Cancer:** Presently bone marrow stem cells are used to help patients following high doses of chemotherapy. Unfortunately the recovered cells are limited in their capacity to restore immune function completely. It is hoped that injection of properly differentiated stem cells would return the complete array of immune response to patients undergoing bone marrow transplants.

**Blindness:** Retinal regeneration with stem cells isolated from the eyes can lead to a possible cure for damaged or diseased eyes and may one day help to reverse blindness.

**Other conditions:** Embryonic stem cells, which can form all types of functional adult cells, provide the hope that such cells can produce the cells or tissues to grow entire hearts, liver and even kidneys, thus solving the problem of the shortfall of organ donors.

**Hair stem cells** have also been isolated and could help people with hair loss by allowing hair cell regeneration.

Recently, new possibilities for the use of adult stem cells have emerged when researchers showed that cells from the bone marrow can give rise to specialized cells in a variety of tissues as different as blood, brain, muscle, kidney, liver and pancreas. One can imagine that in future, we will be able to isolate our own bone marrow cells, treat them and re-introduce them back into the body to renew or repair cells in a number of different organs.

It is hoped that genetic alteration on patient's own bone marrow stem cells and subsequent transplantation, will provide toxicity free transplantation and also the problem of donor scarcity.

### b. Regenerative Medicine

The goal of regenerative medicine is to repair organs or tissues that are damaged by disease, aging or trauma, so that function can be restored or at least removed. Using this definition, most medical acts can be considered as "regenerative" except those that are aimed at prevention of disease such as vaccination.

The term regenerative medicine is used nowadays to describe medical acts, treatments and research that use stem cells to restore the function of organs or tissues. This can be achieved in different ways:

i. By administering stem cells or specific cells that are derived from stem cells in the laboratory.

ii. By administering drugs that coax stem cells that are already present in tissues to more efficiently repair the involved tissue.

### c. Cloning Therapy

An alternative approach to the problem of tissue rejection in organ transplantation is to do the transplantation with cells containing own genetic material. This involves the most contraversial of all stem cell therapies – **therapeutic cloning.**

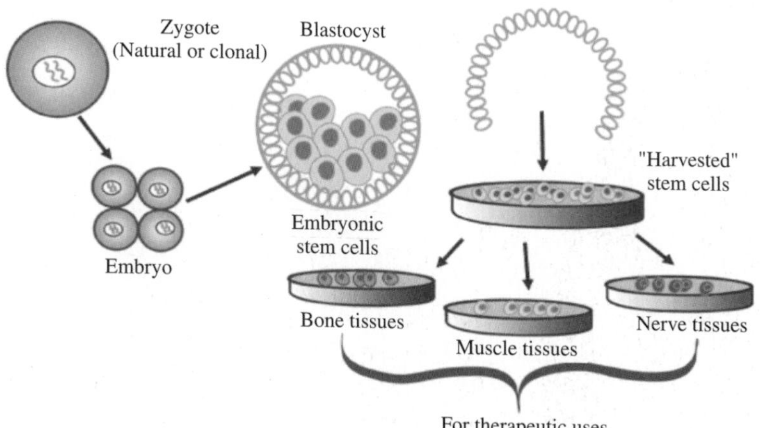


**Fig. 24.2** Proposed model for therapeutic cloning (Source:www.bioethics.ac.uk)

Therapeutic cloning was the intention stated by the US Company, Advanced Cell Technology, when it announced in November 2001, that it had created a cloned human embryo. This was a preliminary development-the longest surviving embryo reached only the six cell stage, and no stem cells were harvested. But, the development was significant because it was done by transferring the nucleus of an adult cell into an egg cell which had its own nucleus removed, called "somatic cell nuclear transfer", this is the same technique that was used to create "Dolly" the sheep. This is used to generate "therapeutic tissues" or "spare organs".

### d. Designer Baby

Advanced reproductive technologies allow parents and doctors to screen embryos for genetic disorders and select healthy embryos. The fear is that in the future it is possible to use genetic technologies to modify embryos and choose desirable or cosmetic characteristics. Designer baby is a term used by journalists to describe this frightening scenario. It is not a term used by scientists.

Advanced reproductive techniques involve using IVF to fertilize eggs with sperm in 'test tubes' outside the mother's body in the laboratory. These techniques allow doctors and parents to reduce the chance that a child will be born with a genetic disorder. At the moment it is only legally possible to carry out two types of advanced reproductive technologies in humans. The first involves choosing the type of sperm that will fertilize an egg: this is used to determine the sex and the genes of the baby. The second technique screens embryos for a genetic disease: only selected embryos are implanted back into the mother's womb. This is called Pre-implantation Genetic diagnosis (PGD).

Recently scientists have made rapid advances in our knowledge of the human genome and in our ability to modify and change genes. In future it may be possible to 'cure' genetic disease in embryos by replacing faulty genes with healthy DNA. This is called germ line therapy and is carried out on an egg, sperm or a fertilized embryo. Such a therapy is successfully been done on animal embryos but at present it is illegal to do this in humans.

CHAPTER 25

# Human Cloning

## INTRODUCTION

Clone is an organism which is genetically an exact replica of another organism. Cloning is to duplicate a cell or an organism usually asexually, which is genetically an exact replica (Xerox copy) of the other cell or organism

Human cloning is the creation of a genetically identical copy of an existing human by non sexual means or growing cloned tissue from that individual. The term is generally used to refer to artificial human cloning.

The following presents the cloning process of how "Dolly" was cloned, and the procedure of how to clone a human. Also presented is a brief outline of the arguments for and against human cloning.

## 25.1 HISTORY OF CLONING

Cloning is totally not a new concept. Experiments with frogs and toads date back to the 1970s. And experiments involving plants and animal embryos have been performed for years. But experiments involving human beings have never been tried or thought possible, until "Dolly." Her birth shocked the scientific community and has spurred discussion about the possibility of human clones. Dr. Lee Silver, a molecular biologist at Princeton University, is optimistic that "human cloning will occur," and that it might take five years, ten years at the outermost. Lee notes that at this time, "no ethical doctor would do human cloning". Although this view is predominant among many scientists, some argue that a safe technology could be developed in the future. This has led to discussion about whether human cloning should even be legally possible.

Numerous events have occurred since the birth of "Dolly" that had only complicated this controversial issue over human cloning.

## Cloning Dolly

- When Ian Wilmut of Roslin Institute, Scotland cloned a sheep, the cloning technique involved somatic cell nuclear transfer in a fully grown mammal, with her DNA coming from a single cell taken from her mother egg, which is fused with the mammary cell. The fused cell then develops into an embryo, which is implanted in a "surrogate" sheep. The embryo grows into a lamb, which is genetically identical to the donor sheep.
- Though has been touted as a success, this cloning procedure is not perfect. It took more than 277 attempts before "Dolly" was created as a health viable lamb. Human cloning is far more complicated, with greater risks and potentials for error. As a result, scientists fear that applying this technique to humans might lead to malformations or diseases in the human clone.

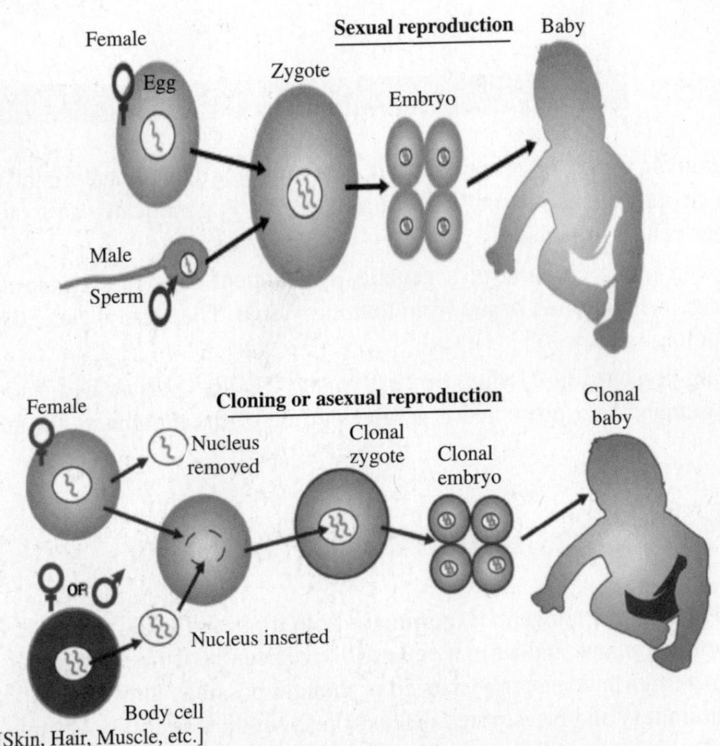


**Fig. 25.1** Figures comparing normal sexual reproduction and asexual reproduction (Source : www.reproductivecloning.net)

- True human cloning would require taking a somatic cell, as opposed to a reproductive cell such as an egg or sperm cell, from a person and removing its nucleus. The DNA of the somatic cell is transferred to an enucleated egg cell. But this is not currently possible because the somatic cells are specialized and there are many genes that have been "turned off" that it is not known how to turn back "on".
- A "**human clone**" is a time-delayed identical twin of another person. A clone is not an exact replica of the original, but just a much younger identical twin. As with identical twins, the clone and the original person will have different fingerprints.

## 25.2 ARGUMENTS FOR AND AGAINST HUMAN CLONING

Human cloning research would enable doctors to determine the cause of spontaneous abortions, give oncologists an understanding of the rapid cell growth of cancer, allow the use of stem cells to regenerate nerve tissues, and advance work on aging, genetics, and medicines.

### Opposition Against Human Cloning

Ian Wilmut, the scientist credited with "Dolly," calls the cloning of humans "appalling," because it would result in a high number of miscarriages and deaths among newborns. A clone could also change family dynamics in profound and unpredictable ways.

The National Bioethics Advisory Commission: "While using animals to understand the biological processes that produced "Dolly" holds great promise for future medical advances, there is no current scientific justification for attempting to produce a human child at this time with this technique".

Concern has been raised that a black market for embryos would arise. Infertile couples could buy a cloned embryo that was stolen or was to be discarded in order to have a child.

Scientists are also concerned about the medical risks and uncertainty associated with human cloning. One fear is that if a baby is cloned, its chromosomes could match the age of the donor-meaning that a "5-year old would look like a 10-year old and a 10-year would look like a 20-year old, with potential for heart disease and cancer to develop".

# Objective Questions

## I. Read the statements and choose the correct answer from the options given

1. Human genetic study encounters problems because
   - i. Individuals are not available for study
   - ii. No techniques are suitable
   - iii. Generation time is too long
   - iv More offspring are produced
   - v. Controlled breeding not possible

   The statements **NOT** applicable to human genetic study are
   - A. i, ii, iii
   - B. i, ii, v
   - C. ii, iii, iv
   - D. iii, iv, v
2. The features of autosomal recessive inheritance are
   - i. Parents of the affected offspring do not express the trait
   - ii. The males will express in higher frequency than females
   - iii. The trait will be revealed in every generation
   - iv. Example for this pattern of inheritance is albinism
   - v. The trait is expressed in both the sexes

   The **correct** statements pertaining to autosomal recessive inheritance are
   - A. i, ii, iii
   - B. i, iii, v
   - C. ii, iii, iv
   - D. i, iv, v
3. The specific features of amniocentesis are
   - i. It is performed when the fetus is 8 weeks old

ii. The sample contains fetus cells only
iii. It is an invasive procedure
iv. It is a therapeutic measure
v. It can detect most of the genetic disease

The statements **NOT** applicable to amniocentesis are

A. i, ii, v
B. iii, iv, v
C. i, ii, iv
D. i, iv, v

4. The features of Hardy Weinberg equilibrium are
   i. It occurs in large population
   ii. The gene frequency fluctuate randomly
   iii. Mating is random
   iv. It is not influenced by mutation and selection
   v. The gene and genotype frequency is constant

   The statements **applicable** to Hardy Weinberg equilibrium are

   A. i, iii, iv
   B. i, iii, v
   C. i, ii, iii
   D. iii, iv, v

5. The features of Kleinfelter syndrome are
   i. Feminized secondary sexual characters
   ii. Presence of one X chromosome
   iii. Occurrence of epicanthal fold
   iv. Gynecomasteia
   v. Infertility

   The statements **applicable** to Kleinfelter syndrome are

   A. i, ii, iii
   B. ii, iv, v
   C. iii, iv, v
   D. i, iv, v

6. Following are some of the technologies applied in human genetics
   i. Somatic cell fusion
   ii. Gamete intra fallopian transfer
   iii. Cytoplasmic transfer
   iv. Karyotype preparation
   v. DNA profiling

Which of the above are **NOT** assisted reproductive technologies?

A. i, iv, v

B. ii, iii, v

C. iii, iv, v

D. i, ii, iii

7. Cancer is produced by

i. Defective DNA repair system

ii. Bacterial infection

iii. High level of enzyme synthesis

iv. Apoptosis initiation

v. Chromosome abnormalities

The statements **applicable** to cancer are

A. ii, iii, iv

B. iii, iv, v

C. i, iv, v

D. i, ii, iii

## II. Match and choose the correct answer

8. With reference to the genetic map construction match the type of maps in Panel I with the technique applied in Panel II and choose the correct option

| I | II |
|---|---|
| 1. Linkage map | a. Somatic cell fusion |
| 2. DNA marker map | b. contig construction |
| 3. Physical map | c. microsatellites |
| 4. cloned fragments | d. LOD score analysis |

A. 1d, 2c, 3b, 4a   B. 1c, 2a, 3d, 4b   C. 1b, 2a, 3d, 4c   D. 1d, 2c, 3a, 4b

9. Match the no of sex chromosome Panel I with the number of Barr bodies given in Panel II and choose the correct option

| I | II |
|---|---|
| 1. XXX | a. Three |
| 2. XO | b. One |
| 3. XX | c. Two |
| 4. XXXX | d. None |

A. 1d, 2a, 3b, 4c   B. 1b, 2c, 3d, 4a   C. 1c, 2a, 3d, 4b   D. 1c, 2d, 3b, 4a

10. Match the mutagen in Panel I with their action given in Panel II and choose the correct option

| I | II |
|---|---|
| 1. gamma rays | a. Depurination |
| 2. acridine dye | b. Deamination |
| 3. ethyl methane sulphonate | c. Chromosome breaks |
| 4. alkylating agent | d. Frame shift |

A. 1b, 2d, 3a, 4c B. 1c, 2d, 3b, 4a C. 1d, 2c, 3b, 4a D. 1b, 2a, 3d, 4c

11. Match the diagnostic test in Panel I with the disease detected given in Panel II and choose the correct option

| I | II |
|---|---|
| 1. Bacterial inhibition assay | a. Cancer |
| 2. Chromosome painting | b. Sickle cell anemia |
| 3. RFLP | c. Individual's identity |
| 4. DNA finger printing | d. Phenylketonuria |

A. 1b, 2d, 3a, 4c B. 1c, 2d, 3b, 4a C. 1d, 2c, 3b, 4a D. 1d, 2a, 3b, 4c

12. Match the disease in Panel I with the symptom given in Panel II and choose the correct option

| I | II |
|---|---|
| 1. Alkaptonuria | a. Scissor walking |
| 2. Cystic fibrosis | b. Sway back posture |
| 3. Lesch nyhan syndrome | c. Salty kisses |
| 4. Muscular dystrophy | d. Black urine |

A. 1b, 2d, 3a, 4c B. 1c, 2d, 3b, 4a C. 1d, 2c, 3a, 4b D. 1d, 2a, 3d, 4c

13. With reference to the Human genome project match the features in Panel I with the appropriate term given in Panel II and choose the correct option

| I | II |
|---|---|
| 1. Largest human gene | a. Transposans |
| 2. Gene dense region | b. Y chromosome |
| 3. Repeated sequences | c. Urban center |
| 4. Less number of genes | d. Dystrophin |

A. 1b, 2d, 3a, 4c B. 1c, 2d, 3b, 4a C. 1d, 2c, 3a, 4b D. 1d, 2a, 3d, 4c

14. Match the mutation mechanism in Panel I with the disease it produces given in Panel II and choose the correct option

| I | II |
|---|---|
| 1. Addition of base pair | a. Huntington disease |
| 2. Base pair substitution | b. Xeroderma pigmentosum |
| 3. Triplet base pair substitution | c. Cystic fibrosis |
| 4. Thymine dimerization | d. Sickle cell anemia |

A. 1b, 2d, 3a, 4c B. 1c, 2d, 3a, 4b C. 1d, 2c, 3b, 4a D. 1d, 2a, 3d, 4c

## III. Read the assertion and reason statements and choose the correct answer from the options given

a. If both the Assertion and the Reason are true statements and the Reason is an adequate explanation for the Assertion.

b. If both the Assertion and the Reason are true statements, but the Reason does not explain the Assertion.

c. If the Assertion is a true statement, but the Reason is a false statement.

d. If both the Assertion and Reason are false statements.

15. **Assertion:** Colour blind sons always have colour blind mother
    **Reason:** The holandric gene in the male is responsible for colour blindness
16. **Assertion:** XIST gene initiates the inactivation of the X chromosome
    **Reason:** The gene is active only in normal female
17. **Assertion:** With regard to stomach cancer the MZ twins and DZ twins show 70% concordance
    **Reason:** A strong role of environment is indicated for stomach cancer
18. **Assertion:** Thalidomide is a teratogen that caused phocomelia
    **Reason:** This is due to the pleiotropic effect of the gene where the gene is not expressed
19. **Assertion:** Telomeres stabilize the chromosome ends
    **Reason:** They form the quadruplex structure
20. **Assertion:** There are regulatory proteins that block the action of enhancers
    **Reason:** They are termed the silencers
21. **Assertion:** In the cell cycle the non-dividing phase is called G1 phase
    **Reason:** There is active DNA synthesis in G1 phase

## IV. Choose the most appropriate answer

22. Human chorionic gonadotropin level in the urine is determined to detect
    a. congenital defects b. pregnancy
    c. chromosomal anomalies d. neural tube defects
23. Haemophilia is sex linked disease that occurs in
    a. males only b. more males
    c. only in females d. equally in males and females
24. Philadelphia chromosome is an example for
    a. Deletion b. Duplication
    c. Inversion d. Translocation
25. Favism and primaquine sensitivity are linked to
    a. Thalassemia b. Cystic fibrosis
    c. G 6 PD defeciency d. Colour blindness
26. Edward syndrome and Patau syndrome are examples for
    a. monosomy b. nullisomy
    c. trisomy d. tetrasomy

27. When a colour blind man marries a normal woman, among the offspring
    a. All the males are colour blind
    b. Only half of the males are colour blind
    c. All the males are normal
    d. Half of the females are colour blind
28. The significant effect of consanguineous mating is
    a. increase in homozygosity
    b. increase in heterozygosity
    c. increase in mutation rate
    d. increase in chromosome anomalies
29. Spina bifida can be best detected by
    a. Ultrasonography
    b. AFP test
    c. Triple test
    d. Fetography
30. Cyclins and kinases are proteins that can
    a. inhibit genes and inhibit cell division
    b. activate genes and activate cell division
    c. inhibit genes and activate cell division
    d. activate genes and inhibit cell division

## Challenging questions

31. Haemophilia is a sex linked recessive trait. A boy has haemophilia and could he have inherited it from the following persons? Justify your answer.
    a. His maternal grand mother
    b. His paternal grand mother
    c. His maternal grand father
    d. His paternal grand father
32. Knowing the concept of origin of cancer by
    i. telomerase expression
    ii. failure of DNA repair mechanism

    How can anti cancer drug be designed?
33. A person with Turner syndrome a mosaic with 45X/46XY. Explain how this mosaicism could arise?
34. A pregnant mother already has a baby with Down syndrome and comes for genetic counseling to you? Sketch out the process of genetic counseling that you will offer.
35. A woman sues a man for support of her child. She has type B blood, her child has O type blood and the man type A blood. Will she win the case? Give your answer with reason.

## Keys to the objective questions:

| | | | | | |
|---|---|---|---|---|---|
| 1. B | 2. D | 3. C | 4. B | 5. D | 6. A |
| 7. C | 8. D | 9. D | 10. B | 11. D | 12. C |
| 13. C | 14. B | 15. d | 16. b | 17. a | 18. c |
| 19. a | 20. c | 21. d | 22. b | 23. b | 24. d |
| 25. c | 26. c | 27. c | 28. a | 29. b | 30. b |

# Glossary

**Acrocentric:** A chromosome with a terminal centromere making one arm very short.

**Achondroplasia:** A form of dwarfism controlled by a dominant gene

**Agammaglobulinemia:** Lack of a class of antibodies impairing immunity

**AIDS:** Aquired Immune Deficiency Syndrome where there is progressive loss of immune function caused by human immunodeficiency virus.

**Albinism:** A genetic disorder marked by the absence of pigmentation.

**Alleles, allelomorphs:** Alternative forms of a gene found in the homologous chromosome.

**Alpha-fetoprotein:** A protein produced by the fetal liver and enters maternal circulation. It's level in the amniotic fluid increases in neural tube defects.

**Alpha thalassemia:** Anemia caused by a mutation in the alpha globin gene

**Amino acid:** Organic molecule with a carboxyl and amino group, which links to other amino acids to form polypeptide chain.

**Amniocentesis:** A method of obtaining fetal cells from amniotic fluid for prenatal diagnosis.

**Amplification:** The production of multiple copies of DNA sequence.

**Ames test:** A simple test that uses bacteria to test chemical compounds for mutagenicity.

**Anaphase:** A stage of cell division, during which chromatids of chromosomes move towards opposite poles of the spindle.

**Aneuploid:** Loss or extra chromosome to a haploid set of chromosomes.

**Antibody:** A protein (immunoglobulin) produced by the plasma cells in response to foreign substance (antigen).

**Anticodon:** A nucleotide triplet in the tRNA complementary to the mRNA codon.

**Antigen:** A foreign substance that stimulates the production of antibody.

**Antisense strand:** The strand of the DNA of a particular gene which is not transcribed into mRNA.

**Artificial insemination:** The technique of placing donated sperm in a woman's reproductive tract.

**Autoimmunity:** Immunity to self due to production of autoantibodies against own antigens.

**Autoradiograph:** An image produced on a photographic film that was placed on a electrophoresis gel and which shows the positions of radioactive molecules in the gel.

**Autosome:** A non-sex chromosome.

**B cells:** Lymphocytes that secrete antibody proteins in response to recognizing non-self molecules.

**Barr body:** A dark stained body representing the condensed, inactivated X chromosome seen in the nuclei of somatic cells.

**Base pair:** A pair of hydrogen bonded DNA bases located between the two backbones of a DNA double helix.

**Base analog:** A kind of mutagen which can mimic the base pairs.

**Benign tumor:** The tumor which does not spread to other parts of the body.

**Beta thalassemia:** Anemia caused by a mutation in the beta globin gene.

**Bivalent:** A pair of homologous chromosomes as seen during metaphase of the first meiotic division.

**Cancer:** A progressive illness caused by uncontrolled cell division.

**Carcinogen:** A substance that causes cancer.

**Carcinogenesis:** A process of cancer development.

**Carrier:** An individual who is heterozygous for a mutant allele.

**Cell cycle:** The sequence of events from one cell division to the other.

**Centromere:** The indented region of a chromosome that divides it into two arms.

**Chiasma:** A cross shaped connection between nonsister chromatids during crossing over.

**Chorionic villus sampling:** A method of obtaining fetal cells for prenatal diagnosis, in which a bit of chorionic tissue is removed from the placenta around $10^{th}$ week of pregnancy.

**Chromatid:** One of the daughter strand of the replicating chromosome.

**Chromosome:** The hereditary vehicle containing genes and located in the nucleus of the eukaryotic cell.

**Chromosomal aberration:** An abnormality of chromosome number and/or structure.

**Chromosome banding:** Staining techniques that give rise to unique pattern of bands in the chromosome.

**Chronic myeloid leukemia:** A type of white blood cell cancer associated with Philadelphia chromosome.

**Cleft palate:** Failure of the bones forming the roof of the mouth to close.

**Clone:** A group of genetically identical cells descended from one cell by repeated division.

**Codon:** A group of three nucleotides in messenger RNA that specifies one particular amino acid.

**Complementary bases:** Nucleotide bases that can pair, purine to pyrimidine by hydrogen bonding.

**Concordant:** The occurrence of a trait in both twins.

**Congenital:** Any abnormality present at birth.

**Consanguineous mating:** Mating between genetically related individuals.

**Cri du chat syndrome:** A deletion in the $5^{th}$ chromosome results in a cat cry in the child.

**Crossing over:** The exchange of chromosome parts between the chromatids of homologous chromosome.

**Cystic fibrosis:** An autosomal recessive disorder caused by the absence of a protein resulting in the formation of thick mucus in the lungs.

**Cytokines:** Immune system biochemicals released from T cells.

**Cytokinesis:** Division of the cytoplasm that occur in telophase stage of cell division.

**Deletion:** Loss of a chromosome segment.

**Denaturation:** Separation of the two strands of DNA in a double helix by breaking the hydrogen bonds between base pairs.

**Deoxyribose:** The sugar that is present in DNA.

**Diabetes mellitus:** Failure of production of insulin leading to a high level of glucose in the blood.

**Dihybrid:** An individual heterozygous for two genes.

**Diploid:** Two sets of chromosomes present in somatic cells.

**Dizygotic twins:** Nonidentical or fraternal twins that arise from two zygotes.

**DNA:** Deoxyribonucleic acid, the genetic material.

**DNA fingerprinting:** A technique for identifying individuals by using DNA probes in electrophoresis.

**DNA hybdridization:** A technique where complementary base pair is used to find out the similarity of genome.

**DNA ligase:** An enzyme that seals two DNA fragments.

**DNA polymerase:** An enzyme that forms a new DNA.

**DNA repair:** A process in which bases that are incorrectly introduced in the DNA are changed to produce the original sequences.

**DNA replication:** Duplication of DNA double helix by using a parental strand.

**Dominant gene:** The allele or phenotype that is expressed even if one allele is present.

**Dosage compensation:** The equalization of expression of X linked genes in both sexes.

**Duchenne muscular dystrophy:** Progressive muscle weakness caused by a sex linked recessive gene.

**Duplication:** An extra segment of chromosome or DNA, resulting in excess dose of genes.

**Ectopic pregnancy:** The implantation of a zygote in the wall of the fallopian tube than in the uterus

**Egg:** The female gamete.

**Electrophoresis:** A technique of separating a mixture of molecules in a paper or gel in an electric field according to their size, shape and electric charge.

**Embryo:** The stage of prenatal development in which organs develop from a three layered organization.

**Embryonic stem cell:** The cell in a mammalian embryo which has not specialized and can be used in gene targeting.

**Empiric risk:** Computation of probability that a trait will occur in a family based on past experience rather than on knowledge of the trait.

**Enhancer:** The DNA sequences that increase the rate of transcription by interacting with promoters.

**Enzyme:** A protein molecule that in small amounts accelerates the rate of chemical reaction.

**Eugenics:** Improvement of human race by encouraging the matings of people with beneficial genes (positive eugenics) and discouraging the matings of people with harmful genes (negative eugenics).

**Eukaryote:** A cell or organism that contains a membrane bounded nucleus with chromosomes.

**Euploid:** The chromosome number that is the exact multiples of haploid number.

**Evolution:** Changes in gene frequency in a population over long period of time that may result in new species.

**Exon:** An expressed coding sequence which is a part of split genes.

**Fallopian tubes:** In a human female, paired tubes leading from near the ovaries to the uterus, where oocytes are fertilized.

**Favism:** Anemia that occurs when a person is deficient of G6PD enzyme and eat fava beans or takes certain drugs.

**$F_1$ generation:** The first generation of offspring from a mating between two parents.

**Fertilization:** Fusion of male and female gamete in sexual reproduction.

**Fetoscopy:** The direct visualization of the fetus in prenatal diagnosis by fetoscope.

**Fingerprint technique:** A method of combining electrophoresis and chromatography to separate the components of a protein.

**Foreign antigen:** A non self molecule that stimulates B cells to manufacture antibodies.

**Fluorescent in situ hybridization (FISH):** A technique in which fluorescent labeled DNA probes are hybridized with the complementary target sequence.

**Frame shift mutation:** A mutation where the reading frame of the gene changes due to deletion or addition of bases.

**Gamete:** A reproductive cell (sperm or ovum).

**Gamete intrafallopian transfer (GIFT):** Reproductive technology in which sperms are transferred from the laboratory to a woman's fallopian tube, where fertilization occurs.

**Gene:** A DNA sequence for the synthesis of a protein.

**Gene amplification:** A technique that uses enzymes of DNA replication in vitro to make many copies of a particular DNA sequence.

**Gene flow:** Movement of alleles between populations.

**Gene frequency:** The proportion of genes in a given population.

**Gene pool:** All the genes present in a population.

**Gene therapy:** Treating a genetic disease by inserting the normal gene.

**Genetic code:** The triplet bases of DNA or mRNA that specify the different amino acids.

**Genetic drift:** Random fixation of genes in a small population.

**Genetic counseling:** Providing guidance to a family regarding the occurrence of a genetic disease and ways to deal with them.

**Genetic screening:** Examining a population for a disease.

**Genome:** The full set of gene in an individual.

**Genotype:** The genetic constitution of an individual.

**Glucose 6 phospate dehydrogenase:** An enzyme involved in aerobic respiration.

**Haploid:** The single set of chromosome.

**Hardy Weinberg law:** In a large randomly mating population, the gene and genotype frequencies remain constant when there is no migration, no mutation, no selection and no genetic drift.

**Heavy chain:** The structural component of an antibody which has high molecular weight.

**Helper cells:** A part of the immune system. This cell has a receptor site which can bind with the MHC and foreign protein.

**Hemizygous:** One allelic condition in a male with regard to X linked genes.

**Hemophilia:** The failure of blood clotting due to the absence of blood clotting factors.

**Heredity:** Transmission of genetic information from parents to offspring.

**Heterogametic sex:** The sex that produces two different kinds of gametes with regard to the sex chromosomes they carry.

**Heterozygous:** The occurrence of two different alleles for a trait present in the same locus in the homologous chromosomes.

**Holandric inheritance:** The inheritance of genes present in the Y chromosome.

**Homogametic sex:** The sex that produces one type of similar gametes with regard to sex chromosomes.

**Homologous chromosomes:** The similar chromosomes are paired one contributed by the father and the other by the mother during fertilization of gametes.

**HLA ( Human leucocyte antigen ):** A specific group of antigens from major histocompatiability complex (MHC).

**Hormone:** A biochemical manufactured in a gland and transported in the blood to a target organ producing a specific effect.

**Human immunodeficiency virus (HIV):** A retrovirus causing AIDS.

**Hybrid:** The offspring of a cross between two genetically different organisms.

**Hydrocephalus:** Swelling of the brain by the accumulation of cerebro spinal fluid.

**Hypertension:** Elevated blood pressure caused by the interactions of genes and environmental factors.

**Immune reaction:** The specific reaction between antigen and antibody.

**Immunogenetics:** The study of the genetic basis of immune system.

**Immunoglobulin:** The antibody.

**Implantation:** Burrying of the fertilized zygote into the uterine wall.

**Inborn error:** A biochemical disorder genetically determined in which absence of a specific enzyme produces a metabolic block.

**Independent assortment:** Mendel's law stating that alleles at different loci on a homologous chromosomes are transmitted independently from generation to generation.

**Infertility:** The inability of a person to produce a child.

**Interferon:** Anti viral protein released by the T cells of the immune system.

**Interleukin:** A class of cytokines that respond to viral infections.

**Interphase:** A part of the cell cycle where there is no cell division.

**Intron:** Intervening sequences that are parts of a gene alternating with exons.

**Inversion:** A type of chromosomal aberrations in which a part of chromosome is broken and reinserted in the reverse order.

**IVF ( In vitro fertilization):** Alternative reproductive technology where the sperm and ovum are allowed to fuse in a glass tube in the laboratory.

**Karyotype:** The orderly arrangement of a chromosome set of a somatic cell.

**Kilobase:** One thousand DNA base pairs.

**Klinefelter syndrome:** An extra X chromosome in a male resulting in abnormalities.

**Law of segregation:** Alleles separate during meiosis.

**Lesch Nyhan syndrome:** Absence of the enzyme HGPRT causes the failure of recycling of the nitrogenous bases of DNA.

**Light chain:** A major structural component of the antibody which has low molecular weight.

**Linkage:** The association between gene present in the same chromosome that they are inherited together.

**Locus:** The position or site of a gene on a chromosome.

**Lymphocyte:** A type of white blood cell produced in the bone marrow that provide immunity.

**Lyon hypothesis:** Refer dosage compensation.

**Malformation:** Morphologic defect due to abnormal development.

**Malignant:** A tumor that is capable of spreading to other tissues in the body.

**Meiosis:** A special type of cell division occurring in gametes resulting in the reduction of chromosome number.

**Memory cells:** B cells which persist after immune response that provides quick response at the next invasion of the same type of antigens.

**Messenger RNA:** The RNA which has complementary sequences for a DNA strand, formed during transcription and functions during translation of a polypeptide.

**Metacentric:** A chromosome with a centrally placed centromere.

**Metaphase:** The stage of a cell division where the chromosomes occupy equatorial plane and have two chromatids each.

**Metastasis:** The spread of malignant tumor cells from one site to other parts of the body.

**MHC:** Major histocompatibility complex (HLA).

**Mitosis:** Somatic cell division resulting in the formation of two daughter cells , each with the same chromosome complement as the parent cell.

**Monoclonal:** Cells that are derived from the same ancestral cell.

**Monoclonal antibody:** A single antibody type produced by hybridoma technology.

**Monosomy:** The condition where there is loss of a chromosome in a set of chromosomes.

**Monozygotic twins:** Twins derived from a single fertilized ovum.

**Multiple alleles:** More than two alleles present in a locus of a chromosome controlling a trait.

**Mutagen:** A substance that induces mutation.

**Mutant:** An individual bearing a mutation.

**Mutation:** Process in which gene or chromosome undergoes changes.

**Neural tube defect:** A birth defect in which part of the spinal cord protrudes due to the failure of closure of the neural tube.

**Non-disjunction:** Failure of separation of homologous chromosomes during cell division.

**Nucleoside:** A purine or pyrimidine base attached to a ribose or deoxy ribose sugar.

**Nucleosome:** A globular unit in a chromatin fibre with a a histone core around which the DNA strand is wound.

**Nucleotide:** A nucleoside attached to a phosphate group.

**Oligonucleotide:** DNA sequence made up of a small number of sequences.

**Oncogene:** A gene that can transform a normal cell into a cancer cell.

**Oocyte:** The female sex cell before it is fertilized.

**Operator gene:** The gene which switches on the structural genes.

**Operon:** A unit of gene function, consisting of an operator gene and structural genes whose action it controls.

**Ovaries:** The paired female reproductive organs which produce eggs.

**Ovulation:** Release of oocytes from the ovary.

**Ovum:** An egg cell.

**Pedigree:** A chart or schematic diagram representing the family history of an individual.

**Pharmacogenetics:** The area of biochemical genetics dealing with genetics of responses to drugs.

**Phenocopy:** The alteration of the phenotype by environmental factors during development which mimics the one that is produced by a gene.

**Phenotype:** The appearance of an individual.

**Phenylketonuria (PKU):** An inborn error of metabolism in which the absence of the enzyme phenylalanine hydroxylase causes impairment in phenylalanine metabolism.

**Philadelphia chromosome:** An aberrant chromosome with a deletion in the long arm of 22 chromosome resulting in chronic myeloid leukemia.

**Placenta:** A specialized organ that connects the developing fetus and the mother.

**Plasma cell:** A mature B lymphocytes which can secrete antibodies.

**Peliotropy:** Many sided effect of a single gene.

**Phocomelia:** Failure of the complete development of limbs.

**Polydactyly:** an autosomal dominant trait characterized by extra fingers and toes.

**Polygenes:** Genes that are present in different loci controlling a trait.

**Polymerase chain reaction (PCR):** A technique that is used to amplify DNA segment.

**Polymorphism:** The occurrence of two or more forms in the same habitat.

**Polypeptide:** A chain of more than one peptide.

**Polyploid:** Multiples of the basic haploid set of chromosomes.

**Population genetics:** Branch of genetics dealing with genetical variation and evolution of a population.

**Porphyria:** An inborn error of metabolism in which a missing enzyme prevents metabolism of red blood cell.

**Prenatal diagnosis:** Techniques employed to diagnose the genetic disease in a fetus before birth.

**Primer:** An oligonucleotide sequence that flanks either side of the DNA to be amplified by PCR.

**Proband or Propositus:** An affected individual who is responsible for identifying the disease in the family.

**Probe:** An artificially synthesized labeled DNA or RNA sequence used to detect the complementary sequence.

**Progeria:** An inherited premature aging disease.

**Promoter:** A DNA sequence that initiates transcription process.

**Prophase:** The first phase of cell division in which the chromosomes become visible.

**Proto oncogene:** A normal gene which when altered can become a oncogene causing cancer.

**Reading frame:** The starting DNA base from which a polypeptide sequence is read.

**Recessive:** A trait which is expressed only in homozygous condition.

**Receptor:** A molecule in or on a cell membrane that has a pocket to fit another molecule triggering chemical activity in a cell.

**Regulator gene:** The gene which controls the rate of synthesis of a product.

**Replication:** The duplication of the double stranded DNA.

**Replication bubble:** The structure formed by the fusion of two replication forks.

**Replication fork:** The structure formed at the site of origin of replication of DNA.

**Restriction endonuclease:** A bacterial enzyme which cleaves the DNA at particular site.

**Restriction fragment length polymorphism (RFLP):** The polymorphism seen in DNA sequence in a population due to the presence or absence of restriction site.

**Restriction site:** A DNA sequence that is cleaved by a specific restriction endonuclease.

**Retinoplastoma:** A rare child eye cancer.

**Reverse transcriptase:** An enzyme that can transcribe RNA into DNA.

**Ribonucleic acid (RNA):** Single stranded nucleic acid having ribose sugar.

**RNA polymerase:** An enzyme that binds to a promoter site and synthesizes mRNA from DNA.

**Schizophrenia:** Loss of ability to perceive leading to aberrant behavior.

**Southern blot:** A technique where DNA fragments run on a electrophoresis is transferred to a nylon membrane and detected by hybridization.

**Spermatogenesis:** The process of formation of sperms.

**Spermiogenesis:** The formation of sperms from spermatids.

**Spontaneous mutation:** A genetic change due to the mispairing.

**SRY:** A gene in the Y chromosome that determines maleness.

**Sub metacentric:** A chromosome having centromere shifted from the centre.

**Surrogate mother:** A woman who carries an unborn child for another woman.

**Syndrome:** A group of symptoms that occur, characterizing a disease.

**Tautomer:** Two forms of a chemical.

**T cells:** Small lymphocytes ( thymus dependent cells ) responsible for cell mediated response to antigens.

**Telomere:** The tip of a chromosome.

**Telophase:** The last phase of cell division resulting in the formation of two daughter cells.

**Teratogen:** A chemical or other environmental agent that causes a birth defect.

**Test cross:** Crossing an individual of unknown genotype to a homozygous recessive individual.

**Testicular feminization:** A male embryo developing female organs though they have XY chromosomes.

**Tissue typing:** Identifying the cell surface protein encoded by genes called HLA complex.

**Transcription:** The formation of mRNA against a DNA template.

**Transition:** A point mutation altering a purine to purine or a pyrimidine to a pyrimidine.

**Translation:** The formation of a protein directed by a specific mRNA.

**Translocation:** A chromosomal aberration involving transfer of a piece of one chromosome to a non homologous chromosome.

**Transversion:** A point mutation altering a purine to a pyrimidine and a pyrimidine to a purine.

**Triplet:** A unit of three linear successive bases in DNA or RNA which codes for a specific amino acid.

**Triple test:** A prenatal test that analyses three substances.

**Trisomy 21:** A extra copy of chromosome 21, causing Down syndrome.

**Tumor suppressor gene:** A gene whose products control normal cell growth and a mutation of this leads to cancer.

**Turner syndrome:** A female with one X chromosome.

**Ultrasonography:** A procedure where ultra sound waves are used to create an image on a video screen. This is often employed in prenatal diagnosis.

**Uterus:** The muscular, sac like organ in the human female in which the fetus develop.

**Wild type:** Allele that is most common for a certain gene in the population producing a normal phenotype.

**Wilms tumor:** A childhood cancer of the kidneys.

**Wilson's disease:** Inability to metabolize copper.

**Xeroderma pigmentosum:** A disorder in which DNA repair is impaired and exposure to sun causes mutations and skin cancer.

**X inactivation:** The turning off of one X chromosome in a female.

**Yeast artificial chromosome (YAC):** A synthesized yeast chromosome capable of carrying large DNA segment.

**Zygote:** The diploid cell resulting from the union of sperm and ovum.

**Zygote intrafallopian transfer (ZIFT):** A technology in which a preembryo fertilized *in vitro* is introduced into the woman's fallopian tube.

# References


Anon. 1997. Human embryo research/fetal experimentation, " Focus on the family and policy statement" @ www.family.org.

Anthony, J.F., William M. Gilbart, Richard, C. Lewontin and Jeffrey H. Miller, 2002. Modern genetic analysis. $2^{nd}$ Ed. W.H. Freeman and Co.

Bhatnagar, Kothari, Mehta. 2002. Essentials of Human Genetics. Orient Longman Ltd.

Dorian J. Pritchard and Bruce R. Korf, 2003. Medical Genetics at a glance. Blackwell Science Ltd.

Elanie Johansen Mangae and Arthur P. Mangae, 1999. Basic human genetics. $2^{nd}$. Ed. Sinaeur Associates. Inc. Sundeland. USA.

Gardner, R.J.M, and G.R. Sunderland, 1996. Chromosome abnormalities and Genetic counseling. Oxford University Press.

Gustavo, Maroni, 2001. Molecular and Genetic analysis of Human traits. Blackwell Science Ltd.

Harold, Vermis. 2001. Stem cell research; Medical progress with responsibility; @ www.doh.gov.uk

Hartl, D.L., 1996. Human genetics. Harper and Row Publishers. New York.

Holland, B. and Kyriacou, C.1993. Genetics and Society. Addison-Wesley.

Jennifer, Gregory, 2001. Applications of genetics. Cambridge University Press.

Knudson Alfred. G. 1971. Mutation and cancer. *Pro. Natl. Acad. Sci*. Vol. 68.

Michael, R. Cummings, 2003. Introduction to Human Genetics. $6^{th}$ Ed. Brooks/Cole Publishers.

Niyogi, A.K. and Srivastava, H.C. 1985. Human Genetics.: Principles and practice. Allied publishers.

Peter Sudbery. 2002. Human Genetics. Pearson and Co.

Pierce Benjamin. A. 1990. The family genetics source book. John Wiley and sons.

Pierce A. Benjamin. 2003. Genetics- a conceptual approach. W.H. Freeman and Company. NY.

Ricki Lewis. 1994. Human genetics and applications. WCB. Publishers. USA.

Salil Basu. 1994. Genetic disorders and health care. Shree Kala Prakashan. New Delhi

Sam Singer.1985. Human Genetics: An Introduction to the principles of Heredity. Freeman and Company. NY.

Tamarin, R.H. 1993. Principles of genetics. 4th Ed. WCB. Oxford.

Thompson and Thompson. 2004. Genetics in medicine. Saunders.

Vincent, M. Ricchardi. 1997. The genetic approach to Human disease. Oxford University Press. NY.

Winston, R, M.C. and A.H. Handyside. 1993. New challenges in human In vitro fertilization. *Science*. Vol. 260 www.genetics-and-society.org

# Index